100 Questions & Answers About HIV and AIDS
Second Edition

Joel Gallant, MD, MPH

Professor of Medicine and Epidemiology
Associate Director, Johns Hopkins AIDS Service
Division of Infectious Diseases
Johns Hopkins University School of Medicine
Baltimore, MD

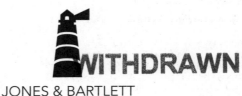

WITHDRAWN

JONES & BARTLETT
L E A R N I N G

World Headquarters
Jones & Bartlett Learning
5 Wall Street
Burlington, MA 01803
978-443-5000
info@jblearning.com
www.jblearning.com

Jones & Bartlett Learning books and products are available through most bookstores and online booksellers.
To contact Jones & Bartlett Learning directly, call 800-832-0034, fax 978-443-8000, or visit our website,
www.jblearning.com.

Substantial discounts on bulk quantities of Jones & Bartlett Learning publications are available to corporations,
professional associations, and other qualified organizations. For details and specific discount information, contact
the special sales department at Jones & Bartlett Learning via the above contact information or send an email to
specialsales@jblearning.com.

Production Credits
Executive Publisher: Christopher Davis
Associate Editor: Laura Burns
Senior Production Editor: Daniel Stone
Marketing Manager: Rebecca Rockel
Manufacturing and Inventory Control Supervisor: Amy
    Bacus
Composition: Abella Publishing Services
Cover Design: Carolyn Downer
Printing and Binding: Edward Brothers Malloy
Cover Printing: Edward Brothers Malloy

Photo Credits
Top left photo: © Nick Stubbs/ShutterStock, Inc.
Top right photo: © Monkey Business Images/
    Shutterstock Inc.
Bottom photo: © Photos.com

The authors, editor, and publisher have made every effort to provide accurate information. However, they are not
responsible for errors, omissions, or for any outcomes related to the use of the contents of this book and take no
responsibility for the use of the products and procedures described. Treatments and side effects described in this book
may not be applicable to all people; likewise, some people may require a dose or experience a side effect that is not
described herein. Drugs and medical devices are discussed that may have limited availability controlled by the Food
and Drug Administration (FDA) for use only in a research study or clinical trial. Research, clinical practice, and
government regulations often change the accepted standard in this field. When consideration is being given to use
of any drug in the clinical setting, the healthcare provider or reader is responsible for determining FDA status of the
drug, reading the package insert, and reviewing prescribing information for the most up-to-date recommendations
on dose, precautions, and contraindications, and determining the appropriate usage for the product. This is especially
important in the case of drugs that are new or seldom used.

Dr. Gallant discloses that as of February 1, 2012, he has had the following financial relationships with
pharmaceutical companies within the prior year:
Research support: Gilead Sciences (paid to Johns Hopkins University)
Consulting fees and scientific advisory boards: Bristol-Myers Squibb, Gilead Sciences, GlaxoSmithKline, Janssen
Therapeutics, Merck & Co., RAPID Pharmaceuticals, Sangamo Biosciences

Library of Congress Cataloging-in-Publication Data
Gallant, Joel E.
    100 questions & answers about HIV and AIDS / Joel Gallant. — 2nd ed.
        p. cm.
    Includes bibliographical references and index.
    ISBN 978-1-4496-5517-4
1. AIDS (Disease)—Miscellanea. 2. AIDS (Disease)—Popular works. 3. HIV infections—Miscellanea. 4. HIV
infections—Popular works. I. Title. II. Title: One hundred questions and answers about HIV and AIDS.
    RC606.64.G35 2013
    616.97'92—dc23
                                    2012002715
6048

Printed in the United States of America
16 15 14 13 12   10 9 8 7 6 5 4 3 2 1

This book is dedicated to Joel Meneses,
my husband, partner, and friend, who has
made my life richer and more joyful.

The author and publisher would like to gratefully acknowledge the contribution of Mike Willis and Rose Ramroop, two patients with HIV infection who have generously shared their experience, insights, and coping tips. Throughout this book, Mike's comments and Rose's comments provide what we hope and expect will be valuable "insider" information for readers from two individuals who are living successfully with HIV infection. Thank you, Mike and Rose.

Mike Willis lives and works in Baltimore, Maryland. He is an advocate for people with HIV disease at Chase-Brexton Health Services and is a musician in his spare time. His medication credo is: "If you can't adhere, at least comply!"

Rose Ramroop lives in Baltimore. She has worked at Johns Hopkins University for 17 years and is now an HIV Counselor for the Johns Hopkins Women's HIV Program. She has served on the Baltimore Ryan White Planning Council and is a member of the advisory board for the Antiretroviral Pregnancy Registry. She has spoken nationally and internationally about HIV in women and children. She is the proud mother of four beautiful girls and spends her free time enjoying life with her family.

CONTENTS

Part 1: Now That You Know   *1*

Questions 1–6 provide information for people who've just been diagnosed with HIV infection, including:

- What's my prognosis?
- Can I live a normal life? What about sex and relationships?
- Who should I tell?
- Should I keep working?

Part 2: The Basics   *11*

Questions 7–14 tell you what you need to know about HIV, your immune system, and the disease in order to understand your condition, your healthcare provider, your treatment options, and how to live with HIV infection. Questions include:

- What's the difference between HIV and AIDS?
- How is HIV spread?
- How can HIV infection be prevented?
- Why isn't there a cure?

Part 3: Diagnosis   *23*

Questions 15–17 are written for people who haven't been diagnosed. Questions include:

- How is HIV infection diagnosed?
- How do I know if I've been recently infected?
- What if all of my tests are negative but I'm sure I'm infected?

Part 4: Medical Care   *27*

Questions 18–21 provide information on finding and paying for medical care, including:

- How do I find the right medical care?
- What are my provider's responsibilities and what are mine?
- How do I deal with my healthcare provider?
- How will I pay for treatment?

Contents

It is very difficult to live among people you love and hold back from offering them advice.

–Anne Tyler, *Celestial Navigation*, 1974

More than 30 years into the HIV epidemic, there is an enormous amount of information available for both patients and clinicians on HIV and AIDS. With web sites and textbooks and pamphlets galore, one would wonder if there is a need for another book about AIDS. I would argue that now more than ever, we need to help our patients take the time to ask and find answers to all of their questions about preventing and living with HIV. In this era of managed care and 15-minute medical visits, there is never enough time to do justice to all of the questions that anyone diagnosed with HIV needs to be asking. *100 Questions and Answers about HIV and AIDS* is a tremendous resource for people living with HIV, their friends, family members, and for healthcare providers. Joel Gallant, a thoughtful and seasoned HIV provider who has been on the frontlines of HIV care for nearly two decades, has done a wonderful job framing the questions that arise from the moment of an HIV diagnosis through the many aspects of living a full life with HIV. Joel's practical, concise, and supportive answers to a wide range of questions help guide the reader through the process of adapting to an HIV diagnosis, getting into care, and making informed decisions for years to come.

—Judith Currier, MD
Professor of Medicine
Chief, Division of Infectious Diseases
Associate Director, UCLA Center for
Clinical AIDS Research and Education
David Geffen School of Medicine at
University of California, Los Angeles

ACKNOWLEDGMENTS

I am indebted to many colleagues and friends, including Jean Anderson, Adriana Andrade, Michael Becketts, Todd Brown, Joseph Cofrancesco, Jeanne Marrazzo, and George Siberry, who reviewed sections of this book, provided valuable feedback, and found important errors. I am especially grateful to Roy Gulick, Jo Leslie, Michael Willis, and to my mother, Donna Gallant, each of whom reviewed the entire manuscript and offered invaluable suggestions. Mary Beth Hansen's comprehensive critique of the manuscript ultimately made this a far better and more useful book. Finally, I thank my patients, who teach me something new every day.

I've been working in the field of HIV/AIDS since the beginning of the epidemic, having started my medical education at "Ground Zero"—San Francisco in 1981. My story will seem like ancient history to those of you who are too young to remember a time without AIDS, but we need history to teach us where we've been and how far we've come. My first patient on my first rotation as a student at San Francisco General Hospital was a terrified young gay man with *Pneumocystis* pneumonia whom I admitted to the world's first AIDS ward on the day it opened. As a terrified young gay man myself, I didn't fully appreciate the historical significance of that day—I was too preoccupied by my own fear. I had come out in the late '70s, when we thought the worst thing you could get from sex was herpes, and condoms were weird things that straight guys wore to keep women from getting pregnant. I knew I was at high risk for the same disease that was killing the men I admitted to the ward. In each young man I cared for, I saw myself and my future, making it hard to appreciate the intellectual challenges or historical significance of what I was learning and experiencing.

At that time in my life, I couldn't face the thought of a medical career devoted to caring for dying gay men, so in a naïve attempt to escape the plague, I left San Francisco in 1985 and moved to New Haven, Connecticut to do the next phase of my training, my medical internship and residency, at Yale. I hadn't escaped, of course, but in New Haven I saw a very different epidemic, one affecting not only gay men but also drug users, heterosexual women, and their children.

There were glimmers of hope during the mid- to late-'80s. HIV was discovered as the cause of AIDS, and a blood test became available. AZT, which prevented death in early studies, was quickly approved. But AIDS remained a devastating, fatal disease that continued to expand its reach both within the United States and throughout the world. During my residency, I spent time working in hospitals in Haiti and sub-Saharan Africa. HIV testing wasn't available there at the time, but the virus made its presence felt in every clinic and on every hospital ward.

At some point during my residency, I realized that the reality of being HIV-positive couldn't be much worse than the anxiety I was experiencing by not knowing my status. When I finally learned I was negative after so many years of fear and uncertainty, things suddenly looked different. Now I could take care of people with HIV without being forced to confront my own mortality on a daily basis. Although there were detours along the way, I ultimately ended up at Johns Hopkins University, where I've been treating people with HIV infection, teaching other clinicians about HIV treatment, and doing research on HIV therapy for more than 20 years.

In the mid-90s, HIV infection was quickly transformed from a progressive, almost universally fatal illness to the chronic, manageable disease that it is today. The speed at which this transformation took place is unprecedented in medical history. However, HIV infection is still a serious, life-altering, and sometimes life-threatening disease.

HIV infection is unique among medical diseases. It's sexually transmitted, has caused the world's largest global epidemic, appeared only in the late 20th century, affects people who are marginalized or discriminated against, carries enormous social stigma, and has completely transformed the world we live in. This book deals primarily with medical issues, but it's impossible to discuss HIV without also talking about relationships, sex and sexuality, mental health, substance abuse, politics, and even about our place in the world and our responsibility to our fellow human beings. Whether we're dealing with HIV infection as patients, clinicians, researchers, or policymakers, we must always view HIV as both a disease that affects individuals and as an epidemic that affects societies.

ACT-UP coined the phrase "Knowledge = Power." In my experience, the people who have the most power over their disease are the ones who educate themselves, seek out expert medical care, adhere to therapy, and optimize the other aspects of their health. *100 Questions & Answers About HIV and*

AIDS is not the definitive book on the subject by any means—there are other books and resources that provide more in-depth and detailed information. Instead, I hope it will serve as a starting point for people with HIV infection—and for those who care about them—one that answers the questions that my own patients ask me, in language that's easy to understand. I hope this book will be the beginning of a long educational journey and that it will help you move from a position of fear to one of knowledge and power.

—Joel Gallant, MD, MPH

Introduction

xvii

Because of the rapid pace of research and drug development, books about HIV infection can quickly become dated. Much has changed since the first edition of *100 Questions & Answers About HIV and AIDS* was published in 2007. The second edition has been extensively updated to include the following important developments:

- New guidelines and research supporting earlier treatment of HIV infection
- Evidence that untreated HIV infection causes inflammation and immune activation with potential long-term consequences that may include "premature aging"
- Research showing the importance of treating HIV-positive people to prevent transmission, as well as the use of pre-exposure prophylaxis (PrEP) and microbicides by HIV-negative people to prevent infection
- New drugs for the treatment of HIV infection, including new single tablet, once-daily regimens, with updated recommendations for first-line therapy and a new table on advantages and disadvantages of the common initial regimens
- New treatments for hepatitis C coinfection that increase the possibility of cure
- Information on use of the newer vaccines (chickenpox, shingles, HPV) in HIV-positive people
- Updated recommendations on screening for osteoporosis in HIV-positive people
- The impact of changing healthcare economics, including healthcare reform, on HIV care in the United States
- Renewed optimism about someday finding a cure for HIV infection

There are many other updates and revisions that I haven't listed here, especially in the area of antiretroviral therapy. I hope that the second edition of *100 Questions & Answers About HIV and AIDS* will be informative and useful, both to seasoned readers of the first edition and to those just beginning their education.

—Joel Gallant, MD, MPH

PART ONE

Now That You Know

What's my prognosis?

Can I live a normal life? What about sex and relationships?

Who should I tell?

More . . .

1. *What's my prognosis?*

Antiretroviral therapy (ART)
Drug therapy that stops HIV from replicating and improves the function of the immune system.

Highly active antiretroviral therapy (HAART)
Antiretroviral therapy meant to suppress the viral load to undetectable levels, using a combination of several agents to prevent resistance.

Cocktail
A common term for an antiretroviral regimen (combination of antiretroviral drugs).

The development of ART is up there with the discovery of penicillin as one of the most important and effective medical achievements of the 20ᵗʰ century, and treatment keeps getting better in the 21ˢᵗ.

Your prognosis is excellent! HIV infection is not the progressive, fatal illness it was in the '80s and early '90s. The memory of those horrible times, together with the stigma that still surrounds HIV infection, can make learning you're positive harder than it has to be. With the right treatment, HIV infection is now a chronic, manageable disease. If it didn't come with so much emotional, social, and historical baggage, people would react to the diagnosis the way they might if they learned that they had diabetes or rheumatoid arthritis. Granted, these aren't perfect analogies, since you can't transmit diabetes or rheumatoid arthritis to others. On the other hand, treatment for HIV is now easier and more effective than treatment for either of those diseases.

Antiretroviral therapy (ART) is the term we use to describe the medications that stop the virus from replicating (multiplying or reproducing). When I speak of "therapy" in this book, I'm referring to ART. Other terms you'll sometimes hear are **highly active antiretroviral therapy (HAART)**, **combination antiretroviral therapy (cART)**, and the "**cocktail**," terms that distinguish combination therapy from the much less effective one- or two-drug therapy we used in the 1980's and early 1990's. However, since all ART is now HAART and cART, I find easier just to use "ART." By stopping the **replication** of HIV, ART keeps the **immune system**—the system in the body that fights infections and cancers—from being damaged further and allows it to recover. The development of ART is up there with the discovery of penicillin as one of the most important and effective medical achievements of the 20ᵗʰ century, and treatment keeps getting better in the 21ˢᵗ.

ART has completely changed the outlook for people with HIV infection. There is no time limit to the benefits of therapy once you start. If you take your medications faithfully, you can keep HIV in check for life, having to change therapy only because of side effects or because better drugs have come along. If you've just been diagnosed, you should plan on sticking around for a long time, living long enough to die of old age. Don't quit your job and max out your credit cards or you may be in for a rude awakening!

ART hasn't been around long enough for me to promise that your lifespan or the quality of your life will be exactly the same as it would have been if you weren't positive, but I feel comfortable telling my newly diagnosed patients that, together, we can virtually eliminate the possibility that they'll ever die of AIDS.

Rose's comment:
When I was first diagnosed, I thought my life was over, and I would never live to see my kids grow up. I became self-destructive because I thought I had no future. I knew nothing about HIV except what I heard from people in the community. In the news I heard about people facing discrimination and stigma and struggling to stay alive. I assumed that that's how life was going to be for me.

It took 8 years before I was ready to learn about the disease. I also had to learn to respect myself, rather than accepting the image that people in the community had of people like me. I live a normal life now. I work, and I have a wonderful family. I'm open now about my HIV status, and I help other HIV-positive people as a peer counselor.

2. Can I live a normal life? What about sex and relationships?

You can have a normal life. . .with a few adjustments. Compared to someone without any chronic medical conditions, you'll have more medical visits and will take more medications. However, treatment for HIV infection has become much easier than it was in the past. Many of my patients now take just one pill once a day and see me for 20 minutes

Replication
The reproduction or multiplication of an organism, including HIV.

Immune system
The system in the body that fights infection.

Now That You Know

3

two to four times per year. They're busy with work or school, are able to travel, to stay physically active, and to maintain relationships.

The biggest adjustments are often the ones that have to do with your relationships with others. Friends and family members may have to be educated before they can treat you like they did before. Sexual relationships present a special challenge. Current partners, if they're negative, will have to face their own fear of infection, a fear not all relationships survive. Entering into new relationships involves the complex issues of disclosure and the fear of rejection or loss of confidentiality (Question 4).

It may be hard to believe now, but in time HIV infection may be low on your list of daily concerns, having little impact on the life you lead and the decisions you make. Getting to that point takes time, support, and sometimes counseling. You may not feel overwhelmed now, but stick with it. . . it gets better.

3. What do I do now?

At a time like this, the last thing you may think you need is a list of tasks, but there are some important things you should do sooner rather than later, and keeping busy with constructive activities can help you cope with your new diagnosis.

- Notify your contacts. Anyone you might have infected or who might have infected you should be notified immediately. (Questions 4 and 85).
- Find a healthcare provider. Question 18 discusses how to find a provider who has expertise in treating HIV infection.
- Get some lab tests. The most important tests to get right away are the **CD4 count (or CD4 cell count)**, **viral load (or plasma HIV RNA)**, and a **resistance test**, discussed in Part 5.

CD4 count (or CD4 cell count)

A lab test that measures the number of CD4 cells in the blood (expressed as number of cells per cubic millimeter).

Resistance test

A blood test (either a genotype or phenotype) that looks for evidence in the presence of HIV that is resistant to antiretroviral medications.

Viral load (or plasma HIV RNA)

A lab test that measures the amount of HIV RNA in the plasma (blood), expressed as "copies per milliliter."

- Educate yourself. Reading this book is a good start, but don't stop there. You'll find more sources of information in the appendix.
- Think about money. How are you going to pay for care? Do you have insurance? What does it cover? Do you qualify for any benefits on the basis of your HIV infection? If you're not sure, talk to a social worker or case manager (Question 21).
- Get support. Seek out the people in your life who you can talk to about your HIV infection, and tell them. If there aren't any, find a good counselor, therapist, or support group. Don't go through this alone (see Question 4)!

Michael's comment:
After my positive HIV test result, I saw a psychologist. I talked with him for a year before I got up the nerve to tell my family. Now that they know, we get along better, and I see them more often than I did before I was diagnosed. Therapy helped me to become more comfortable with myself. Facing a life-threatening illness brought up all the insecurities I'd ever felt about anything, and having someone outside of my daily life to talk to helped a lot. As my best friend said, "This way you won't run off all your friends."

4. Who should I tell?

Telling people about your HIV status is a big step, especially when you've just found out you're positive. Some people should be told right away; with others, you have time to think it over.

It's important to tell people you might have infected or who might have infected you—sex partners or people you've shared needles with. They need to find out so they can get tested, for their own benefit and to protect others. Your provider, counselor, or case manager may also be able to help you inform partners. If those don't seem like good options, health departments can notify your contacts and advise them to get tested without revealing your name.

Think about telling friends or family members you rely on for emotional support. It's critical to have a support system when dealing with HIV infection. Think about the important people in your life. Will they be there for you? Will they respect your confidentiality? If so, think about telling them. Family members don't need to know just because they're family members. You pose no risk to them, and you may outlive them anyway. You should tell them if they'll be part of your support network.

If you're not comfortable telling friends or family members, then you need to look elsewhere. Ask about support groups, counselors, peer advocates, or therapists in your community. Internet chat groups, while not the best source of reliable medical information, can be helpful places to share your experiences with other HIV-positive people in an anonymous setting.

You should also inform your healthcare providers, including doctors, dentists, counselors, and therapists. They need to know your HIV status to be able to take care of you properly. If you have a provider you don't feel you can tell, then it may be time to change providers.

You *don't* have to tell your boss, your coworkers, your plumber, or the guy sitting next to you on the bus.

> *Michael's comment:*
> Sometimes I had to console the people I chose to tell. I found myself having to take on the supportive role, rather than feeling supported. I also found that no one kept my secret. Be prepared.

Rose's comment:

Be careful who you tell, and tell them carefully. When I was first diagnosed 20 years ago, I told my mother and my youngest sister. They gave me a lot of support in the beginning, but they were afraid to let anyone else find out. My sister told people I would be dead from a brain tumor in 6 months. My mom would only invite me and my kids over when no one else was around. We had to drink out of paper cups, eat off paper plates, and take out our own garbage. When I didn't die in 6 months, my sister start-ing telling people that my daughter and I were positive, thinking she was protecting the community.

Things got better for me when I started speaking publicly about HIV. I talked about the discrimination I faced within my own family. As my family got educated, they became more supportive. They apologized for the way they had treated me, but I still felt angry.

I wound up taking care of my mother when she got cancer. I didn't show my anger because she was dying and I loved her. I wish I'd been treated the same way.

5. Should I keep working?

If you've just been diagnosed with HIV infection but are feel-ing well, you should keep working. You've got a long life ahead of you, and you're going to need the money and insurance, not to mention the opportunity to remain productive and to maintain a sense of purpose.

If you're sick, you may be disabled. Your disability is likely to be temporary if you haven't started ART yet because you'll probably get a lot better once you start therapy. However, HIV infection can also lead to permanent disability despite

Social Security Disability Insurance (SSDI)

A monthly Social Security benefit for disabled people who have worked in the past and have paid a minimum amount of Social Security taxes.

Supplemental Security Income (SSI)

A federal cash assistance program designed to help the aged, blind, and disabled who have little or no income to pay for basic necessities.

Family Medical Leave Act (FMLA)

A federal law that allows people to take time off work without fear of termination or loss of benefits to deal with their own serious or chronic medical problems or those of their family members.

treatment, especially in people with advanced disease or in those who develop severe complications that have long-lasting consequences.

You may qualify for temporary or permanent disability payments either through your employer, private disability insurance, **Social Security Disability Insurance (SSDI)**, or **Supplemental Security Income (SSI)**. Talk to your provider, a social worker, or a case manager about what you might qualify for. If you intend to keep working but expect frequent absences due to illness or medical visits, you should consider filing for benefits under the **Family Medical Leave Act (FMLA)**, which will protect your job and benefits. Information on FMLA is available online or through your employer's human relations department.

Many HIV-positive people are now doing well but qualify for permanent disability because of complications that happened years ago. Some of them aren't working, while others have chosen to give up their disability and go back to work. This can be a tough decision. It's hard to go back to work after years of not working, to explain long gaps in your employment history to a prospective employer, to give up a steady income, and to give up other benefits that often come with being on disability, including Medicaid. On the other hand, disability payments aren't guaranteed for life. Applications have to be renewed frequently, and unless your medical records indicate that you're *currently* disabled, the checks may stop coming someday. If you feel you're able to return to work after a period of time on disability, there are federal and state transition programs that offer return to work programs and benefits. If you're wrestling with this decision, talk it over with your provider, social worker, or case manager.

Michael's comment:
When I was diagnosed, I was sick enough to get SSDI benefits. SSDI stinks. The pay is bad, for one thing. And wait until you meet a prospective partner who asks, "So,

what do you do?" Medicare doesn't kick in until you've been getting SSDI for 2 years, so I didn't have insurance, which was worrisome. When my health improved, I returned to work, and I'm glad I did. Work gives me a sense of purpose. It's fun, and the pay is better. When Mr. Right asked me where I work, I didn't have to look down at my shoes and mumble.

Rose's comment:
Working makes me feel like I'm making a contribution. I'm a part of society and am living a normal life. Not everyone can work, but for me, it's part of my therapy and keeps me alive. My work gives me a goal and a purpose. It's also fun to prove people wrong who told me I'd be too sick to work.

6. But I don't *know!* Should I get tested?

If you're reading this book and asking this question, the answer is *yes!* Routine HIV testing is now recommended for all adults and adolescents, which means that everyone should know his or her HIV status. You could disregard this recommendation if you've never had sex or shared needles, but in general we'd be a lot better off if we stopped worrying about "risk factors" and just tested everybody. We have a simple, cheap, highly accurate test for a disease that's spread from person to person, is highly treatable, and is fatal if untreated. It's a crime that so many people don't get diagnosed until they're really sick.

People sometimes get tested because they're afraid they might have been infected from a specific event. A negative test 3 months after exposure is highly reassuring. To be 100% sure, get another test at 6 months. Better yet, if you're sexually active—and especially if you're having unprotected sex—it makes more sense to get tested routinely every 6 to12 months rather than try to time the test based on the exposure, which can drive you (and your medical provider) crazy.

Routine HIV testing is now recommended for all adults and adolescents, which means that almost everyone should know his or her HIV status.

Sexually transmitted infections (STIs)
Infections transmitted from person to person through sexual activity.

Hepatitis B
A viral infection of the liver caused by hepatitis B virus (HBV).

Hepatitis C

A viral infection of the liver caused by hepatitis C virus (HCV).

Tuberculosis (TB)

A bacterial disease caused by *Mycobacterium tuberculosis*.

Shingles (herpes zoster)

A painful, blistering rash, usually occurring in a band on one side of the body, caused by reactivation of the chickenpox virus (varicella zoster virus, VZV).

Lymphoma

A type of cancer involving cells of the immune system, called lymphocytes.

Thrombocytopenia

Disorder in which there is an abnormally low amount of platelets.

Anemia

A condition in which the body does not have enough healthy red blood cells.

Leukopenia

A decrease in the number of white blood cells found in blood.

Having just recommended that everyone get tested, it seems redundant to list other reasons for testing, but here goes. Testing is *especially* recommended for people who've had **sexually transmitted infections (STIs), hepatitis B, hepatitis C, tuberculosis (TB), shingles (herpes zoster),** or problems that could be caused by HIV infection, such as weight loss or chronic diarrhea. HIV testing should be performed in anyone with **lymphoma,** or unexplained **thrombocytopenia** (low platelet count), **anemia** (low red blood cell count) or **leukopenia** (low white blood cell count). All pregnant women should be tested since treatment can prevent transmission to their infants.

PART TWO

The Basics

What's the difference between HIV and AIDS?

How is HIV spread?

How can HIV infection be prevented?

More . . .

HIV

The abbreviation for human immunodeficiency virus, the virus that causes HIV infection and AIDS.

AIDS

Acquired immunodeficiency syndrome, a more advanced stage of HIV infection, defined by having a CD4 count below 200 or one of a list of AIDS indicator conditions.

Life cycle

In HIV infection, the stages that the virus goes through, starting with its entry into human cells and ending with its replication and the release of new virus particles into the blood.

Retrovirus

A virus that contains RNA and that can turn RNA into DNA through reverse transcription using viral enzymes.

Enzymes

Proteins that carry out a biological function.

RNA

Ribonucleic acid, the genetic material of the HIV virus.

7. What is HIV?

HIV stands for "Human Immunodeficiency Virus." It's the virus that causes **AIDS** (Acquired Immunodeficiency Syndrome). The difference between HIV infection and AIDS is discussed in Question 10. HIV is passed from person to person through sexual contact, blood exposure, childbirth, and breastfeeding (Question 12).

It's time to take a brief detour into the basic science of the **life cycle** of HIV—I promise to make it short. For even more details, see Question 29. Refer to **Figure 1** since a picture will make this easier to understand. HIV is a **retrovirus**, a virus that contains **enzymes** (proteins) that can turn **RNA**, its genetic material, into **DNA**. It's called a retrovirus because this is the reverse of the normal sequence in which DNA is converted (through the process of **transcription**) into RNA. After infection, HIV RNA gets turned into DNA by the **reverse transcriptase** enzyme. The DNA is then inserted into the DNA of human cells. That DNA can then either be used to create new viruses, which infect new cells, or it can remain latent in long-lived cells (**reservoirs**), such as **resting CD4 cells**. HIV's ability to remain latent is what allows it to persist for life, even with effective treatment. It's what has kept us from finding a cure so far (Question 14).

When it's not treated, HIV infection causes progressive damage to the **immune system** and is almost universally fatal. It is the world's most serious **pandemic** (global **epidemic**), and there are no immediate prospects for either a cure or a preventive **vaccine**. Fortunately, treatment today is highly effective, and deaths from HIV disease are now mostly preventable in countries where therapy is available and affordable.

8. Where did HIV come from?

Research now shows that **HIV-1***, the most common kind of HIV worldwide, first infected humans in sub-Saharan

*HIV-2 is a related but much less common virus found mostly in West Africa.

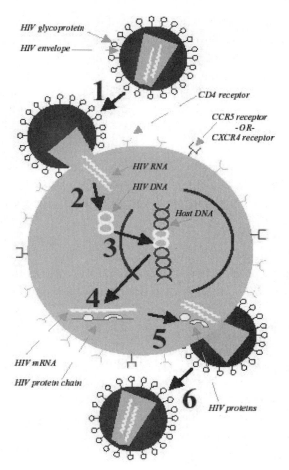

DNA

Deoxyribonucleic acid, the genetic material of humans and most other life forms.

Transcription

The process of turning DNA into RNA.

Reverse transcriptase

An enzyme contained within the HIV virus that can turn viral RNA into DNA so it can be inserted into the DNA of human cells.

Latency

The ability of HIV to persist in human cells for the lifetime of an infected individual by inserting its DNA into long-lived reservoir cells.

Reservoirs

Long-lived human cells that can be infected by HIV, allowing it to persist (remain latent) for the lifetime of the individual.

Vaccine (vaccination)

A substance that is given, usually by injection, but sometimes by mouth or by nasal spray, to stimulate the immune system to make antibodies against a bacterial or viral pathogen.

Figure 1

1. **Entry:** CD4 attachment, coreceptor finding, and fusion. HIV begins its life cycle when it attaches to a CD4 receptor and then binds to one of two co-receptors (CR5 or CXCR4) on the surface of the CD4 cell. The envelope (coating) of the virus then fuses with the CD4 cell. After fusion, the virus inserts its RNA (genetic material) into the host cell.
2. **Reverse Transcription:** An HIV enzyme (protein) called reverse transcriptase converts the RNA of the virus into HIV DNA.
3. **Integration:** The newly formed HIV DNA enters the nucleus of the CD4 cell, where an HIV enzyme called integrase inserts it into the human DNA of the CD4 cell. The DNA of the virus can remain hidden for many years in resting CD4 cells, or can be used to create new virus in activated CD4 cells.
4. **Transcription and translation:** In an activated CD4 cell, the HIV DNA is transcribed into RNA, which is then translated into HIV proteins.
5. **Assembly:** An HIV enzyme called protease cuts long chains of HIV proteins into smaller individual proteins. New virus particles are assembled from the smaller HIV proteins and copies of HIV RNA.
6. **Budding:** The newly assembled virus buds (pushes out) from the CD4 cell. The new copies of HIV are now free to infect other cells.

Adapted with permission from AIDSinfo, an HHS information service managed by NIH.

Resting CD4 cells

CD4 cells that live a long time and can harbor HIV DNA, which can't be affected by antiretroviral therapy because it's not replicating. An important reservoir of latent HIV.

Epidemic

The appearance of new cases of disease (especially an infectious disease) in a human population at a higher rate than would be expected.

Pandemic

A global epidemic.

HIV-1

The most common form of HIV worldwide.

HIV causes illness mainly by damaging the immune system.

CD4 lymphocyte (or CD4 cell, or T-helper cell)

A type of lymphocyte (a type of white blood cell) that can be infected by HIV. CD4 cells fight certain infections and cancers.

White blood cell (WBC)

A type of blood cell that helps fight infection.

Africa at some point in the first half of the 20th century. It was transmitted from chimpanzees, probably when people came into contact with their blood while hunting or butchering. HIV probably remained confined to Africa for many years, in part because travel within and from Africa was uncommon then. We have definite proof of human infection with HIV in Africa dating back to 1959.

The virus eventually spread beyond Africa, probably entering the United States in the mid- to late-70s. Unusual cases of rare infections and cancers began to be seen in gay and bisexual men between 1979 and 1981, and the AIDS epidemic is said to have begun in 1981, when these reports first appeared in medical journals, making it clear that there was an emerging epidemic. The HIV virus was discovered in 1983, leading to a blood test and eventually to treatment.

The disease was originally reported in gay and bisexual men, but the "risk groups" were later expanded to include injection drug users, hemophiliacs, and Haitians. It eventually became clear that "risk behaviors" were more important than "risk groups." People could be infected through unprotected sex, exposure to infected blood, or through labor or breastfeeding. It's now estimated that over 33 million children and adults were infected with HIV worldwide as of the end of 2009.

9. How does HIV make you sick?

HIV causes illness mainly by damaging the immune system. It can infect many human cells, but the most important target is the **CD4 lymphocyte** (also known as the **CD4 cell** or **T-helper cell**). The CD4 cell is a type of **white blood cell (WBC)** that is responsible for controlling or preventing infection with many common viruses, bacteria, fungi, and parasites, as well as some cancers. HIV infection leads to destruction of CD4 cells. Over time, the number of CD4 cells (the CD4 count) declines. Although it may take years, the CD4 count eventually becomes so low that there aren't enough cells to fight certain infections or cancers, which allows symptoms or complications to occur. The speed at which the CD4 count falls varies from person to person and depends on a number of factors, including genetic characteristics, characteristics of the viral strain, and the amount of virus in the blood (viral load).

The reason for the loss of CD4 cells still isn't completely understood. It's not simply a matter of HIV infecting and directly killing the cells, because the proportion of cells that are actually infected is small. We now know that HIV infection causes a chronic **immune activation** (stimulation of the immune system), which may be responsible for the reduction in the number of CD4 cells. Chronic inflammation may also increase the long-term risk of certain medical conditions, such as coronary heart disease or cancers (see Questions 28 and 63).

In addition to damaging the immune system, HIV can directly affect many of the body's organs, such as the nervous system (Question 73) and the kidneys (Question 49). It can also cause weight loss, night sweats, and diarrhea (Question 11). When deaths due to AIDS were common, it was often said that people didn't die of HIV itself, but of one of its complications, such as a cancer or infection. While that may have been technically true in most cases, HIV infection was still the underlying problem that led to death from AIDS.

10. What's the difference between HIV and AIDS?

Everyone who has AIDS has HIV infection, but not everyone with HIV infection has AIDS. AIDS stands for acquired immunodeficiency syndrome. It's "acquired" because you only get it by being infected with HIV from someone else who has it. "**Immunodeficiency**" means it causes damage to the immune system. It's a "**syndrome**" because in the years before HIV was discovered and identified as the cause of AIDS, we recognized a collection of symptoms and complications, including infections and cancers that occurred in people who had common risk factors.

HIV infection leads to destruction of CD4 cells.

Immune activation

A general stimulation of the immune system that can be caused by a variety of infections, including HIV infection. In the case of HIV, it is thought to cause the decline in CD4 count that occurs with time.

Immunodeficiency (or immunosuppression)

A state in which the immune system is damaged or impaired, either from birth (congenital immunodeficiency) or acquired, as in HIV infection.

Syndrome

A collection of signs or symptoms that frequently occur together but that may or may not be caused by a single disease.

Opportunistic infection

An infection that takes advantage of immuno-deficiency.

The term AIDS was coined in 1982. HIV hadn't been discovered yet, so there was no way to know whether people were sick until they were truly sick. Someone was said to have AIDS if he (and it was mostly men in those days) developed one of a long list of **opportunistic infections (OIs)** and cancers that don't occur in people with healthy immune systems (Question 53). After HIV was discovered and a test became available, the definition of AIDS changed so that being HIV-positive was required. In 1993, the **Centers for Disease Control and Prevention (CDC)** expanded the definition of AIDS to include people with CD4 counts of less than 200. The current **AIDS case definition** is shown in **Table 1**.

Avoid the term "full-blown AIDS." It's old-fashioned, unnecessarily scary, and doesn't mean anything other than AIDS. In fact, the term AIDS isn't all that useful either. If you're HIV-positive, the disease you have is **HIV infection (or HIV disease)**. AIDS just refers to a more advanced stage of that disease. Treatment can prevent HIV infection from turning into AIDS, and it can restore the health of people with AIDS. In the eyes of the organizations and scientists who keep track of the epidemic, once you have AIDS, you'll always have AIDS. But what matters more to your provider—and what should matter more to you—is how you're doing *now*.

11. What are the stages of HIV infection?

The first stage of HIV infection, occurring a few weeks after transmission, is called **primary HIV infection** or **acute retroviral syndrome (ARS)** (Question 16). During ARS, standard HIV tests (**serologies**) are sometimes negative, but the amount of virus in the blood (measured by the viral load) is extremely high, making it easy to transmit HIV to others.

ARS resolves on its own and is followed by a latent stage usually called **asymptomatic HIV infection**. People generally feel fine during that stage, although their **lymph nodes** may be enlarged (**lymphadenopathy**), and some common conditions

Table 1   AIDS Indicator Conditions (CDC AIDS Case Definition, 1993)

- Candidal esophagitis [64*] (or candidiasis of the respiratory tract, which is rare)
- Cervical cancer, invasive [61,80]
- Coccidioidomycosis involving an organ other than the lungs [57]
- Cryptococcosis involving an organ other than the lungs [57]
- Cryptosporidiosis with diarrhea for at least 1 month [65,91]
- CMV disease involving an organ other than the liver, spleen, or lymph nodes [58]
- Herpes simplex with ulcers lasting more than 1 month [88] or with esophagitis [64] or infection of the respiratory tract (rare)
- Histoplasmosis involving an organ other than the lungs [57]
- HIV-associated dementia [72]
- Isosporiasis (a parasitic disease that is uncommon in the United States) with diarrhea for at least 1 month [65]
- Kaposi's sarcoma [61]
- Lymphoma [61]
- Mycobacterium avium complex (MAC) [55], Mycobacterium kansasii, or other mycobacterial infection involving organs other than the lungs
- Tuberculosis [59]
- Pneumocystis pneumonia (PCP) [54]
- Pneumonia, bacterial: two or more episodes in 1 year [66]
- Progressive multifocal leukoencephalopathy (PML) [71,72]
- Salmonella with bloodstream infection, recurrent [65]
- Toxoplasmosis [56]
- Wasting syndrome (greater than 10% weight loss plus chronic diarrhea, weakness, or fever lasting more than 30 days) [68]

*Numbers in brackets refer to questions in which the topics are discussed.

can occur more often or be more severe, including vaginal yeast infections, herpes, or shingles.

Some people develop symptoms of HIV infection before actually developing AIDS. This stage is referred to as **symptomatic HIV infection** (formerly **AIDS-related complex**, or **ARC**). Symptoms include weight loss, oral **thrush** (a **yeast** infection in the mouth), persistent diarrhea, night sweats, and fatigue.

You have AIDS if your CD4 count falls below 200 (whether or not you have symptoms) or when an **AIDS-indicator condition** (or **AIDS-defining condition**) has been diagnosed (see Table 1). Most people reach a CD4 count of 200 before

Acute retroviral syndrome (ARS)

A collection of symptoms, such as fever, rash, and swollen lymph nodes, which most people experience during primary infection, shortly after they're infected.

Serologies

Blood tests that measure antibodies to look for evidence of a disease.

Asymptomatic HIV infection

An early stage of HIV infection in which infected people have a positive test but no symptoms.

Lymph nodes

Structures of the human body that are part of the immune system, acting as filters that collect and destroy bacteria and viruses.

You have AIDS if your CD4 count falls below 200 or when an AIDS-indicator condition has been diagnosed.

The Basics

Lymphadenopathy

Swollen or enlarged lymph nodes ("glands").

Symptomatic HIV infection

A stage of HIV infection in which people have symptoms caused by HIV, such as weight loss, diarrhea, or thrush, but have not yet developed an AIDS indicator condition.

AIDS-related complex (ARC)

An old term, no longer in use, for the stage of HIV disease in which people have symptoms but have not yet developed AIDS.

Thrush

Oral candidiasis, a yeast infection involving the mouth presenting with white/yellow curd-like plaques on the palate, gums, or the back of the throat.

Yeast

A group of micro-organisms (that can sometimes cause human infections, ranging from minor (oral thrush, vaginitis) to severe (cryptococcal meningitis).

developing complications, so a low CD4 count is the most common reason for an AIDS diagnosis. As the CD4 count declines further, the list of possible complications grows. We sometimes refer to someone with a CD4 count below 50 as having **advanced HIV infection**.

If it's not diagnosed and treated, HIV infection almost always progresses from early stages to late stages, eventually resulting in death. Treatment can move you from a late stage to an early stage. Having AIDS or advanced HIV infection is not a good thing, but HIV infection is treatable at any stage.

12. How is HIV spread?

There are only a few ways in which HIV can be spread.

- *Sexual transmission.* For HIV to be spread through sex, the semen, vaginal fluids, or blood of an infected person must enter the body of an uninfected person. This usually happens through vaginal or anal intercourse. The risk is greatest if the "insertive" partner (the one "on top") is positive, but the person on top can be infected by the one on the bottom, too. HIV can also be transmitted by oral sex, if infected semen, vaginal fluids, or menstrual blood get in the mouth. (For a more detailed discussion of reducing sexual risk, see Questions 13 and 86.)
- *Blood exposure.* HIV can be transmitted through transfusion, though the risk is virtually non-existent in places where the blood supply is tested. Far more commonly, it's transmitted through injection drug use, when negative users share needles or syringes ("works") with positive users. Healthcare workers have been infected when they've been stuck with needles containing infected blood or when their eyes, nose, or open cuts have been splashed with blood or body fluids from an HIV-positive patient.
- *Childbirth and breastfeeding.* HIV-infected women can pass HIV to their infants during childbirth (usually at the time of labor or shortly before) or by breastfeeding (see Question 76). Infants aren't infected at the time of

conception, so an HIV-positive man can only infect the infant indirectly by infecting the mother.

HIV isn't spread through contact with saliva, urine, sweat, or feces, and contrary to popular belief, it is *not* transmitted by mosquitoes, exposure of body fluids to intact skin, holding hands, kissing, hugging, sharing drinking glasses or eating utensils, mutual masturbation, or having naughty thoughts!

13. *How can HIV infection be prevented?*

HIV is an entirely preventable disease. The means of prevention are directly related to the modes of transmission (see Question 12).

- *Sexual transmission, HIV-negative people.* It doesn't get any safer than abstinence. But while this approach has its vocal supporters, it's not acceptable to everyone, and even among the most virtuous, sometimes "sex happens." The next best alternatives are to (1) limit the number of sexual partners, (2) engage in sexual activities other than anal or vaginal intercourse, (3) use condoms when you *do* have intercourse, and (4) avoid getting semen, pre-seminal fluid ("pre-cum"), and vaginal fluids in your mouth or eyes. For more details on safer sexual practices, see Question 86. HIV-negative people should play it safe regardless of what they're told about their partners' status. Partners don't always know or reveal their current status or their status may change. If you're HIV-negative and engaging in frequent unprotected sex, you might also want to consider pre-exposure prophylaxis (PrEP), which involves taking certain antiretroviral medications to prevent transmission. This is a new approach that isn't being widely practiced yet, but studies show it's effective when the medications are taken regularly. Less clear is how it will be implemented and paid for. It may be an option for some, especially those with insurance who have providers who are knowledgeable about ART and PrEP. Another

AIDS indicator condition (or AIDS-defining condition)
One of a list of conditions, including opportunistic infections and malignancies, that is used by the CDC to determine who has AIDS.

Advanced HIV infection
The most advanced stage of HIV infection, usually in people with CD4 counts below 50 or 100.

The Basics

new approach is the use of vaginal or rectal microbicide (virus-killing) gels, used as lubricants before intercourse. These are being studied and are at least partially effective, but aren't available as of this writing.

- *Sexual transmission, HIV-positive people.* If you're HIV-positive, it's your responsibility to never infect anyone else (regardless of the behavior or preferences of your partners). Condoms are effective when used regularly and correctly, but they don't work when left unopened in the nightstand drawer. Even more important than condoms is being on effective ART with an undetectable viral load (Questions 28 and 86), which is the most important way for positive people to avoid infecting others.

- *Drug use.* The best way to prevent infection from drug use is to get treatment and stop using. But if you're going to use drugs, don't share needles and syringes. That can be easier said than done, especially in backward places that don't have needle exchange programs. If you have to share syringes and needles, decontaminate them with bleach.

- *Transmission to infants.* All pregnant women should be tested for HIV infection. Treatment during pregnancy is almost 100% effective at preventing transmission to the baby (Question 76). HIV-positive women should not breastfeed their babies.

If no one shared needles and everyone wore condoms during sex, the HIV epidemic would disappear.

Don't spend time worrying about obscure ways of transmitting the virus. The simple fact is that if no one shared needles and everyone wore condoms during sex, the HIV epidemic would disappear.

14. Why isn't there a cure?

Given how long the disease has been around, it may seem strange that science hasn't come close to finding a cure for HIV infection. Conspiracy theorists argue that a cure exists but is being suppressed by profit-motivated drug companies or by evil governments trying to cull their populations of less desirable elements. I'll leave that discussion for later (see Part 16), and I'll talk about science here.

It may surprise you to learn that there is only one viral disease that has ever been cured with medical treatment—hepatitis C. All other viral diseases either kill you quickly (Ebola virus), get better on their own (the common cold), remain dormant in your body forever (herpes), or are preventable with vaccination (measles). The fact that HIV hides out in the DNA of long-lived human cells makes it an especially difficult problem to tackle.

It's also worth noting that most of the other diseases that we suffer from in the developed world are also chronic, incurable, but treatable diseases. Think of diabetes, high blood pressure, coronary artery disease, heart failure, arthritis—none of them curable, all of them manageable (though not always as easily manageable as HIV infection).

Since writing the first edition of this book, I've become more optimistic about the possibility of a cure. You may have heard about the Berlin patient, an HIV-positive man with leukemia who appears to have been cured of HIV after getting a bone marrow transplant using bone marrow from a donor who was genetically immune to HIV infection. This is not the cure we've been looking for. Bone marrow transplants are expensive and dangerous procedures, and people who get them require lifelong immunosuppression to prevent rejection. But the Berlin patient tells us that cure is possible, and his experience may lead to safer ways to achieve this goal. Alternatively, we could develop a "functional cure:" a treatment that doesn't eliminate HIV from the body, but that allows the immune system to keep it under control without ART. Cure and eradication research is now a high priority at the NIH. Provided that we continue to generously fund scientific research (not necessarily a safe assumption these days), the search for a cure will be the focus of some of our best scientists.

The Basics

In about 15 years, we saw HIV infection go from being an almost universally fatal, untreatable illness to a manageable, chronic disease.

In the meantime, it would be a mistake to look at cure as the only measure of success. In about 15 years, we saw HIV infection go from being an almost universally fatal, untreatable illness to a manageable, chronic disease and treatment became easier and better in the 15 years that followed. A cure will be a scientific breakthrough of unprecedented proportions; until then, we'll have to be content with triumphant, unparalleled success.

PART THREE

Diagnosis

How is HIV infection diagnosed?

How do I know if I've been recently infected?

What if all of my tests are negative but
I'm sure that I'm infected?

More . . .

Enzyme-linked immunoassay (EIA or ELISA)

The initial antibody test used to diagnose HIV infection.

Western blot (WB)

The confirmatory test used to diagnose HIV infection in people who test positive for HIV antibodies by ELISA.

Indeterminate HIV serology

This occurs when the EIA is positive but the Western blot contains some bands that are seen with HIV infection, though not enough to make a diagnosis.

Seroconversion

The process of developing an antibody to an infectious agent.

Antibodies

Proteins used by the immune system to fight infection.

Antigens

Proteins from organisms, such as bacteria or viruses, that stimulate an immune response.

Window period

The period between infection and formation of antibodies leading to a positive HIV test (serology).

15. How is HIV infection diagnosed?

If you already know you're positive, you can skip this section, which was written for readers who don't know their status or who have questions about testing.

Tests to diagnose HIV infection are highly accurate. With the standard blood test (serology), the lab first does an **enzyme-linked immunoassay (ELISA** or **EIA)**. A negative ELISA generally means you're not infected, though it can be negative if you've been infected very recently. If it's positive, the lab automatically runs a second test called a **Western blot (WB)**. If both tests are positive, you're infected. False positives tests are extremely rare. When they happen, it's usually due to a clerical error: a mislabeled tube or the wrong name on the lab report.

Sometimes the ELISA is positive and the WB is indeterminate—not completely negative but not fully positive either. An **indeterminate HIV serology** can occur for one of two reasons. First, you might have been recently infected and are in the process of **seroconversion** (development of a positive serology), in which case a repeat test will soon be fully positive, usually within 1 month. Second, you might be negative but just happen to have an indeterminate test for reasons that will probably never be determined. If the test remains indeterminate for 1 to 3 months and you have an undetectable viral load, you're not infected.

The serology can be negative if you've just been infected. Most people who are infected develop **antibodies** within 2 to 8 weeks; 97% are positive within 3 months and 100% within 6 months. The newer fourth generation HIV tests, which detect both HIV antibodies and **antigens** (proteins on the surface of the virus), can detect HIV earlier, shortening the **"window period"** by 1 to 2 weeks. Viral load testing (HIV RNA) is sometimes used to diagnose recent infection, and a very high viral load always indicates infection. But a viral load is not a perfect diagnostic test because it can be negative (**undetectable**) in people who are infected, and it can be positive (**detectable**) at low levels in people who aren't infected. It *is* a useful test to diagnose acute retroviral syndrome in people with symptoms (Question 16).

Rapid tests can give you a result within a few minutes, using either blood or saliva. **Home tests** (see *Home Access* at www .homeaccess.com/) can be mailed in, and results are given over the phone. These tests are accurate if they're negative, but a positive test should always be confirmed with a standard serology.

16. How do I know if I've been recently infected?

Most people feel sick within a few weeks of HIV infection. This is called primary infection or acute retroviral syndrome (ARS) (Question 11). The illness may be mild and brief or it may be severe enough to require hospitalization. In most cases, the symptoms are similar to those of the flu or mononucleosis. They can include fever, muscle aches, fatigue, sore throat, swollen lymph nodes, or rash. Less often, people can develop neurological symptoms, such as **Bell's palsy** (paralysis of one side of the face), **aseptic meningitis**, **Guillain-Barré syndrome** (paralysis that starts in the legs and moves up the body), or **myopathy** (muscle pain and weakness). Sometimes, people with ARS become seriously immunosuppressed and develop opportunistic infections that normally occur only in people with longstanding HIV disease, but this happens rarely.

During ARS, the standard HIV test (serology) may be negative or indeterminate, though fourth generation antibody/ antigen tests are likely to be positive. The viral load will be very high (in the hundreds of thousands or even millions). If the serology is negative and the viral load is undetectable, then HIV is not the cause of the symptoms.

Unfortunately, the diagnosis of ARS is often missed. The symptoms are nonspecific (common to other viral conditions), and many healthcare providers don't think about ARS or don't

Diagnosis

Undetectable

A term used to describe a viral load that is too low to be measured by a viral load test.

Detectable

A word used to describe a viral load that is high enough to be measured by a viral load test.

Rapid tests

HIV tests that provide an answer within a few minutes, using either blood or saliva.

Home tests

An HIV blood test that can be used at home.

Bell's palsy

A paralysis of one side of the face that can be caused by a variety of infections, including acute HIV infection.

Aseptic meningitis

Meningitis that is not caused by a bacterium that can be grown in culture.

Guillain-Barré syndrome

Progressive muscle paralysis starting in the legs and moving upward, sometimes seen during acute retroviral syndrome.

Myopathy

An inflammation of muscles causing muscle pain and weakness, sometimes seen with acute retroviral syndrome, high-dose zidovudine, or "statins" used to lower cholesterol.

Clinical trial

A study in which a treatment for a medical condition is tested in human volunteers to determine the safety and/or effectiveness of the treatment. (See Glossary for types of clinical trials.)

HIV is not hard to diagnose.

---

know how to diagnosis it. It's important to diagnose HIV infection at this stage for several reasons. First, people with ARS have enormous amounts of HIV in their blood, semen, and vaginal fluids. They can easily spread HIV to others if they don't know they're infected. Second, it's possible to be infected with drug-resistant HIV (virus that isn't suppressed by one or more drugs). The best time to test for transmitted resistance is during ARS (Questions 16 and 24). Finally, there may be a benefit to starting treatment during ARS. This hasn't been proven, but it's a reason for people with ARS to consider being treated or joining a clinical trial.

17. What if all of my tests are negative but I'm sure that I'm infected?

I don't want to come down too hard on the "Worried Well"—people who are convinced they have HIV infection despite overwhelming evidence to the contrary. After all, I'm hoping they'll buy so many copies of this book that we'll have to print more for the folks who really have HIV. But the simple fact is that HIV is not hard to diagnose. If the serology is negative 6 months after your last exposure, you're negative. You don't need a viral load, a DNA test, or a viral culture. You don't need to see a specialist. You don't need to think about rare subtypes, or whether medications you take are causing false negative tests results.

What you *may* need is a psychiatrist or a psychotherapist. Irrational obsession with disease can be a sign of depression, obsessive-compulsive disorder, or hypochondriasis. Depression and anxiety can cause many of the symptoms that lead the Worried Well to think they're infected. People may also obsess about HIV infection because it's easier than dealing with more difficult issues like guilt or anxiety about sexuality or infidelity.

My advice: Put this book down (after you buy it), stay off the Internet, and start addressing the underlying causes for your concern about HIV infection.

PART FOUR

Medical Care

How do I find the right medical care?

What are my provider's responsibilities
and what are mine?

How will I pay for medical care?

More . . .

18. How do I find the right medical care?

People treated by HIV experts stay healthier and live longer than those managed by non-experts.

The choice of a medical provider may be the most important one you make so make it carefully. Treating HIV infection is complex; it's not something that should be attempted by providers without experience and training. Studies have shown that people treated by HIV experts stay healthier and live longer than those managed by non-experts. Mistakes made by inexperienced clinicians early in the course of therapy can lead to drug resistance that never goes away. I know of doctors who will refer their patients to dermatologists for zits, but who will try to manage HIV by themselves. Don't let that happen to you! If your doctor says he hasn't managed many HIV-positive patients, but "it can't be that hard," run away!

I use the term "expert," because there's technically no such thing as an "HIV specialist." An HIV expert is simply a clinician with lots of HIV experience who keeps up with the latest research on therapy. Some infectious disease specialists are HIV experts, but some aren't. There are general internists and family practitioners who *are* HIV experts. Experts don't even have to be doctors. There are expert nurse practitioners and physician assistants, which is why I tend to use terms like "clinician" or "healthcare provider" rather than "doctor" in this book.

Case manager

A person who helps coordinate your medical care, provides referrals for needed services, and determines whether you qualify for any assistance or entitlement programs.

AIDS service organization

An organization that provides services to people with HIV infection.

Finding expert care can be tricky. If you have a primary medical provider, he or she may be able to refer you to someone. Ask a **case manager** or someone at an **AIDS service organization** for a recommendation. Talk to infected friends or support group members. Look for an expert in your area on the web site for the American Academy of HIV Medicine (www.aahivm.org) or the HIV Medicine Association (www.hivma.org).

Having HIV doesn't mean you have to give up your primary provider. Some HIV experts serve only as consultants to primary providers, while others provide primary medical care to their positive patients. What matters is that your HIV care be directed by an expert, and that the expert and your primary provider communicate with each other.

As I write this, the future of expert HIV care is unknown. Fewer healthcare providers are choosing HIV medicine as a career, and as healthcare reform takes effect, many people who now get their care in Ryan White-funded HIV specialty clinics may have to move to primary care clinics that don't have the same level of expertise or support services. In an ideal world, everyone would have an HIV expert managing their care, but I can't promise that everyone will always have access to that kind of expertise.

19. How do I deal with my healthcare provider?

The provider who treats you for HIV infection is going to be an important person in your life for a long time. This is someone you should like, trust, respect, and be able to communicate with. As with any long-term relationship, the first may not be "The One." Don't be afraid to shop around. Here are a few questions you should ask when you start a relationship with a new provider:

1. *Are you covered by my insurance plan?* This question is usually answered by the office staff or by someone from your insurance company before you ever see the provider.
2. *How much experience do you have? How do you keep up with the latest advances in the field?* These are awkward questions, but only someone who doesn't have what it takes will answer them defensively. You should have a sense of your provider's level of experience and how he or she keeps up with new developments in the field.
3. *Will you be my primary provider or will you act as a consultant? Who should I contact about urgent medical problems?* The answer to the questions may be up to you, the provider, or your insurance company, but it's important to clarify them early on.
4. *How often will I see you? When do I get lab work drawn—before the visit or on the same day?* Either is fine, but personally I find that having recent lab results available at the time of the appointment makes for a more productive visit.

5. *How do I reach you between visits for questions, new problems, or emergencies?* Some providers use e-mail to communicate with patients; others have special phone-in hours; others use nurses, physician assistants, or nurse practitioners for first contact. Find out who covers your provider for questions and emergencies when the provider is not on call.

6. *Where would I go if I needed to be hospitalized?* You'd like to think that a great provider would be affiliated with a great hospital, but it doesn't always work that way. Make sure you'd be comfortable going to the hospital your provider admits patients to.

20. What are my provider's responsibilities and what are mine?

Since your relationship with your provider should be a partnership, there are mutual responsibilities that both parties should be aware of.

Your Provider's Responsibilities

1. To treat you with respect and to pay attention to your concerns and opinions.
2. To ensure that urgent medical care is available to you at all times.
3. To keep you informed about your health status, your progress, and your prognosis in language you can understand.
4. To tell you about your treatment options and to be willing to provide advice about which option he or she thinks is best.
5. To inform you of important side effects or long-term toxicities of medications and to help you weigh the risks and benefits of therapy (without overwhelming you with a long list of bad things that rarely happen).

Your Responsibilities

1. To treat the provider and staff with respect.
2. To provide a complete history, even if it means tracking down old medical records yourself. Better yet, keep your own records! See **Table 2** for a list of things you should keep track of.
3. To keep appointments or to cancel them with plenty of notice whenever possible.
4. To follow the course of treatment agreed on and to let the provider know about problems early so that treatment can be changed.
5. To be honest about what's going on in your life and with your treatment... even if it means disappointing your provider.

Michael's comment:
When I showed up at Dr. Gallant's office, I was a lot sicker than I realized. My CD4 count was in the double digits and my viral load was sky-high. I was losing sensation from the waist down. I'd only been infected for about a year and a half and was a fast progressor. What allowed me to live was:

1. *Medicines that work.*
2. *A doctor who knows what he's doing. (He is the author of this book, after all!)*
3. *Following the treatment plan that I agree to.*

21. How will I pay for medical care?

Because this book is written from a U.S. perspective, the answer is complex. We don't really have a "healthcare system" in this country—not yet anyway. What you're entitled to depends on who you are, whether and where you work, and where you live. That being said, *most* people who need HIV care in the United States have been able to get it. Having HIV

Table 2 Information to Keep Track of and Share with New Providers

Dates
- Date of HIV diagnosis
- Approximate date of infection, if known (dates of exposure, previous negative tests, acute retroviral syndrome, etc.)
- Dates of major complications

Test results (with dates)
- CD4 counts
- Viral loads
- Resistance tests (genotypes and phenotypes)
- Hepatitis A, B, and C serologies
- *Toxoplasma* IgG antibody
- CMV IgG antibody
- Syphilis tests
- Gonorrhea and chlamydia tests
- Pap smears (cervical and/or anal)
- Tests for latent TB infection (tuberculin skin test or interferon-gamma releasing assay)
- Other tests, if applicable (HLA B*5701, tropism assay, etc.)

Vaccinations (with dates)
- Tetanus (dT or Tdap)
- Pneumococcal (Pneumovax)
- Hepatitis A
- Hepatitis B
- Influenza (flu)
- Travel vaccines

Treatment history
- All antiretroviral therapy (with start and stop dates for each drug)
- Side effects and allergic reactions
- Prophylaxis or treatment for opportunistic infections or complications

Other important information
- Emergency contacts
- Case manager or social worker
- Advance Directives (living will, Durable Power of Attorney for Health Care)

A year's worth of ART costs between $12,000 and $22,000 per year, not including medical visits or lab tests. Few people pay for this out of pocket.

infection entitles you to benefits that would not be available if you had some other disease. It's a far cry from universal health care, but we take what we can get!

HIV care is expensive. A year's worth of ART costs between $12,000 and $22,000 per year, not including medical visits or lab tests. Few people pay for this out of pocket. Those with private insurance are generally covered, though some insurance plans require high co-pays or have limits on medication coverage that can be exceeded long before end of the year. There may be programs that can help cover these costs; talk to your case manager or social worker.

If you're uninsured, or if your insurance doesn't cover your medications, you may qualify for the **AIDS Drug Assistance Program (ADAP)** in your state. This is a program that provides HIV medications to people who fall below a specified income level. The coverage provided by ADAP programs varies from state to state. Some states' programs are quite generous, whereas others* are skimpier and may have waiting lists or shorter lists of covered medications. Medical visits and lab tests are often paid for by federal **Ryan White Care Act** funds that are received by some HIV providers or treatment centers. As I write this, Ryan White funding remains intact, but its future is uncertain, as I've discussed in Question 18. Finally, people with HIV infection may qualify for **Medicaid** or **Medicare**, depending on income, assets, and the degree of disability.

The complexities of insurance, benefits, and entitlements vary too much and change too quickly for me to be able to do justice to them in this book. My advice is to talk to an HIV-savvy case manager or social worker, and find out where you stand. You can find a case manager or social worker at HIV clinics and AIDS service organizations.

AIDS Drug Assistance Program (ADAP)

A federally funded program that provides antiretroviral medications and other HIV-related medications to those who have no other way to pay for them.

*I won't name names, but they know who they are!

Ryan White Care Act

A government-funded program that provides money on a state or local level to provide care for uninsured people with HIV infection.

Medicaid

An insurance program funded by the federal and state governments that provides coverage for medical care to low-income, uninsured people.

Medicare

A federally funded program to provide medical insurance primarily to the elderly and disabled.

Medical Care

PART FIVE

X

Getting
Started

What does my CD4 count mean?

What is a resistance test, and when should I get one?

What vaccinations do I need?

More . . .

Red blood cell (RBC)

A blood cell that carries oxygen to the organs of the body.

Platelet

A blood cell that helps blood clot.

Lymphocyte

A type of infection-fighting white blood cell. CD4 cells are a type of lymphocyte.

Prophylaxis

Prevention, usually applied to the use of medications taken to prevent opportunistic infections or to keep them from coming back after they've been treated.

CD4 percent

The percentage of lymphocytes that are CD4 cells.

CD8 cells (or CD8 lymphocytes, or T-suppressor cells)

Another type of lymphocyte affected by HIV infection.

Viral load

A lab test that measures the amount of HIV RNA in the plasma (blood), expressed as "copies per milliliter."

Log (logarithm)

Another way of expressing viral load results.

22. What does my CD4 mean?

Your blood contains **red blood cells (RBCs)**, white blood cells (WBCs), and **platelets**. **Lymphocytes** are a type of WBC, and the CD4 cell is a specific type of lymphocyte, the one most affected by HIV. The CD4 count measures the health of your immune system. It should be checked regularly (usually every 3 to 6 months) if you're not on therapy because it measures the amount of damage done by HIV and is the most important test for deciding whether you need to start ART (Question 28) or **prophylaxis** (prevention) for opportunistic infections (Question 60). The CD4 count almost always increases with effective ART, but how much it will increase is hard to predict.

Once you're on ART, the viral load becomes more important than the CD4 count as a measure of your response. If your viral load is undetectable—the goal of therapy—it's unlikely that you would make any changes based on the CD4 count. An ideal response to ART is to have an undetectable viral load and a CD4 count that's above 500. When you reach that goal, it's not necessary to measure the CD4 count more than once a year.

The CD4 count can vary from day to day—even from hour to hour. It can drop temporarily when you're sick or have been vaccinated and can be affected by the way it's processed in the lab. Don't pay too much attention to a single count, and don't get too worried (or excited, for that matter) about a single count that's not consistent with previous counts. It's the *trend* that matters, not one number. When in doubt, you can also look at the **CD4 percent**—the percentage of your lymphocytes that are CD4 cells. This number doesn't vary as much as the CD4 count, so if your CD4 count has changed but your CD4 percent hasn't, chances are it's not a real change. And once your CD4 count is normal (above 500), don't worry about changes within the normal range. Normal is normal. If it's 650 once, 710 next, and 580 after that, those are all great results.

CD8 cells (or **CD8 lymphocytes,** or **T-suppressor cells**) are also affected by HIV infection, but it's not necessary to measure them, since we don't use the CD8 count or the CD4/CD8 ratio to make treatment decisions.

23. What's a viral load?

The viral load (viral HIV RNA) measures the amount of HIV in your blood. It's a measure of the activity of the virus and of how well ART is working. It's also used, along with the CD4 count, to help decide whether to start treatment.

The viral load can range from very low (less than 20 to 75 copies per milliliter of blood) to very high (millions of copies). It is highest during the acute retroviral syndrome and in people with advanced disease who aren't on treatment. When treatment is effective, the viral load should be undetectable—less than 20 to 75, depending on which lab test you're using. Having an undetectable viral load doesn't mean there's no virus; it just means that the viral load is too low to be measured by standard blood tests.

Your viral load should be measured routinely (usually every 3 to 4 months). Regular measurements are especially important once you start treatment because that's how you know whether the drugs are working. If you've been on ART with an undetectable viral load for many years, getting it checked every 6 months is sufficient. The viral load should drop at least ten-fold [1 **log (logarithm)**] during the first month of therapy (e.g., from 100,000 to 10,000), and it should be undetectable within 3 to 6 months, depending on how high it was before you started.

Getting Started

Blip

A single detectable viral load with undetectable viral loads before and after.

Failure

Loss of activity of ART. Includes virologic failure (detectable viral load on therapy), immunologic failure (falling CD4 count on therapy), and clinical failure (worsening symptoms on therapy).

Resistance

The ability of the virus to replicate despite the presence of antiretroviral medications.

Genotype

In HIV, a type of resistance test that looks for specific resistance mutations known to cause resistance to antiretroviral drugs.

Phenotype

A type of resistance test that measures the ability of the virus to replicate in varying concentrations of antiretroviral drugs.

Mutations

Changes in the normal genetic make-up of an organism due to a mistake that occurs during reproduction.

If your viral load is detectable once in a while, don't panic. It may just be a "**blip**"—a single viral load that's detectable at low levels (below 1,000). Blips can result from normal lab variation (no lab test is 100% accurate), so they usually don't amount to anything. The current definition of treatment failure is a viral load of above 200 that's been repeated and confirmed. Of course, you can't be sure it's a blip until you repeat the test, which is important to do, since a detectable viral load can also be a sign of early treatment **failure**.

24. What is a resistance test, and when should I get one?

Resistance tests tell you which drugs your virus is resistant to. Not all viruses respond to all medications. Resistance tests help your provider choose the best drugs to treat your virus.

Unlike CD4 counts and viral loads, resistance tests aren't ordered on a regular basis. They're ordered for only two reasons: to find out whether you were infected with resistant virus and to find out whether you've developed resistance if your treatment is failing. You should be tested for resistance as soon as possible after you're diagnosed with HIV, even if you're not starting ART right away. The test becomes less accurate if it's delayed. Your provider should also order a resistance test if you're failing therapy, to determine which drugs are no longer working and which drugs to use next.

There are two types of resistance tests—**genotypes** and **phenotypes.** Genotypes look for **mutations** (changes) on the genes of the virus that cause resistance to specific drugs. Phenotypes measure the virus's ability to replicate (multiply or reproduce) in the presence of drugs. Genotypes are faster and cheaper, but they can be hard to interpret if there are a lot of mutations. Phenotypes take longer and cost more, but they measure resistance more directly and are better at determining whether a drug still has partial activity despite mutations.

Resistance tests aren't perfect. The lab may not be able to do the test if your viral load is below 1,000, and the tests are better at finding out which drugs *won't* work than which ones *will*. Bad news (evidence of resistance) is always believable, but you have to take good news (evidence of sensitivity to drugs) with a grain of salt. They can't always give you reliable information about drugs you've taken in the past, because resistant virus may be present but no longer detectable. Don't ignore old resistance test results. If resistance was detected 5 years ago, it's still there—even if it doesn't show up now on the test.

25. What other tests do I need?

Here's a list of important tests. Some are ordered just once when you're first diagnosed, while others are ordered on a regular basis:

- **Complete blood count (CBC)**. Every 3 to 6 months to look for anemia (**hemoglobin** and **hematocrit**), low white blood cell count, or platelet problems.
- **Comprehensive chemistry panel.** Every 3 to 6 months to assess the liver, and kidneys, among other things.
- **Hepatitis tests.** Baseline testing for hepatitis A, B, and C and follow-up antibodies for A and B after vaccination to see if the vaccines worked (Questions 79 and 80). If the initial tests show evidence of either chronic hepatitis B or C, then you need further testing, including hepatitis B or C viral loads tests (**HBV DNA** or **HCV RNA**).
- **Tests for sexually transmitted infection.** Tests for **syphilis**, **gonorrhea**, and **chlamydia** at least once a year if you've been sexually active (Question 88).

Getting Started

HCV RNA

The "viral load" for hepatitis C, used to confirm the diagnosis in people with a positive HCV antibody, to make the diagnosis in some people with a negative antibody, and to monitor response to hepatitis C therapy.

Tuberculin skin test [TST or purified protein derivative (PPD)]

A skin test used to look for evidence of past exposure to the TB bacterium.

Interferon-gamma releasing assay (IGRA)

A blood test used to detect latent infection with the TB bacterium as an alternative to a tuberculin skin test.

Toxoplasmosis

Disease caused by the parasite, *Toxoplasma*.

Pap smear

A diagnostic test used to look for cervical dysplasia and cervical cancer.

Cervical dysplasia

Abnormal cells of the cervix, the mouth of the uterus, caused by human papillomavirus (HPV).

- **Tuberculosis testing**. **Tuberculin skin test (TST,** or **purified protein derivative [PPD])** or **interferon-gamma releasing assay (IGRA)**, to find out whether you've been exposed to the bacterium that causes **tuberculosis** (Question 59).
- **Toxoplasma IgG antibody**. To find out whether you've been exposed to the parasite that causes **toxoplasmosis** (Question 56).
- **Pap smear**. In women, to look for **cervical dysplasia** (changes in the cells of the cervix) or cancer. Pap smears should be repeated at least yearly. **Anal pap smears** should also be considered in both women and men, especially those who've had receptive anal sex (Question 81).
- **Fasting glucose and lipid panel**. Before starting antiretroviral therapy and periodically after that, especially if you're on HIV drugs that increase cholesterol, triglycerides, and blood sugar (Question 43).
- **Urinalysis**. To look for kidney problems or signs of infection (Question 49).

Other tests that are sometimes ordered include antibodies against CMV (anti-CMV IgG), a chest x-ray, and an HLA B*5701 assay, to find out whether it's safe to take abacavir (see Question 45).

26. What vaccinations do I need?

- **Tetanus toxoid (dT or Tdap)**. You need a booster every 10 years whether you're HIV-positive or not.
- **Pneumococcal polysaccharide vaccine (*Pneumovax*)**. This helps protect you against **pneumococcus**, a bacterium that causes pneumonia. One booster after 5 years is recommended.
- **Hepatitis A vaccine**. If you've never had **hepatitis A** and you're not immune to it (with a positive total or IgG **HAV antibody**), consider getting the two-shot vaccine series with follow-up antibody testing to be sure the vaccine

worked. Hepatitis A vaccine is especially important for people with chronic hepatitis B or C.

- **Hepatitis B vaccine.** If you've never had hepatitis B and you're not immune to it with a positive surface **(HBsAb)** antibody, you should get the three-part vaccine series with follow-up antibody testing to be sure the vaccine worked. There's also a three-dose combination vaccine (*Twinrix*) that protects you against both hepatitis A and B.

- **Influenza ("flu") vaccine.** A flu shot is recommended in the fall, not because HIV-positive people get more flu or worse flu than anyone else, but because it's a drag to get the flu*. Get the injectable vaccine, not the live virus nasal spray.

- **Varicella (chickenpox) vaccine.** If your CD4 count is above 200, you've never had chickenpox or shingles and you have a negative anti-varicella IgG antibody, consider getting this vaccine.

- **Shingles (herpes zoster) vaccine.** Not yet approved for HIV+ people, but consider it if you're over 60 and have a CD4 count above 200.

- **Human papillomavirus (HPV) vaccine.** Not yet approved for HIV-positive people, and most are already infected with HPV, but it can be considered, especially in young men and women.

Vaccines for international travel are discussed in Question 93.

Vaccines work best when the immune system is strong. If you'll soon be starting ART, now may not be the best time to get vaccinated. The vaccines will be more effective if you wait until after your CD4 count has risen and your viral load is undetectable.

*The flu vaccine cannot *cause* the flu. It's given during cold season, so it's inevitable that some people will catch a cold shortly after getting vaccinated and will blame the vaccine. Don't be one of those people!

HAV antibody
A blood test for hepatitis A.

HBsAb (or anti-HBs)
A blood test for hepatitis B.

Influenza ("flu")
A viral infection caused by influenza virus that causes fever, muscle aches, respiratory symptoms, and gastrointestinal symptoms.

Varicella (chickenpox)
The virus that causes chicken pox and shingles (herpes zoster).

Shingles (herpes zoster)
A painful, blistering rash caused by reactivation of the chickenpox virus.

Human papillomavirus (HPV)
A sexually transmitted virus that causes abnormal cells (dysplasia) in the cervix, anus, and mouth, which can lead to cancer if not treated.

Getting Started

PART SIX

Starting Treatment

How does antiretroviral therapy work?

How do my provider and I choose my first regimen?

Why is adherence so important?

More . . .

27. How does antiretroviral therapy work?

Antiretroviral drugs don't kill HIV; they stop it from replicating (reproducing itself). If you stop replication, you stop the virus from infecting new cells. Suppressing replication also reduces the immune activation and inflammation that are thought to cause much of the damage to the immune system (Question 9). Turning off replication, immune activation and inflammation allows the immune system to recover and the CD4 count to increase.

Combination therapy has been a guiding principle since the mid-90s. The reason for combining several drugs into a single **regimen** or "cocktail" is to prevent resistance. When the virus reproduces, it makes mistakes. These mistakes are called mutations. Billions of **virions** (virus particles) are produced each day if you're not on therapy. Because of the high error rate, almost every mutation that *could* occur *does* occur, on a daily basis. Before the days of HAART, treatment for HIV involved a combination of one or two relatively weak drugs. Mutations that allowed the virus to replicate in the presence of those drugs could appear spontaneously. Those resistant mutants then had an advantage over the original **wild-type virus** (drug sensitive virus without mutations). Over time they became selected as the predominant **strain**, and the drugs were no longer effective.

However, it's far more difficult for the virus to spontaneously develop enough mutations to cause resistance to multiple drugs. When you're taking an ART regimen that includes several active drugs, resistance can only occur when drug levels aren't high enough to keep the virus from replicating, such as when you miss doses.

While most current ART regimens consist of at least three drugs, there's probably nothing magic about the number three. It may be possible to use fewer drugs if they're potent and if the virus needs several mutations to become resistant to them.

Combination therapy

The use of more than one antiretroviral drug to suppress HIV infection.

Antiretroviral drugs don't kill HIV; they stop it from replicating (reproducing itself).

Regimen

A combination of antiretroviral drugs.

Virions

Single virus particles.

Wild-type virus

The strain of HIV that occurs "in the wild"—without the presence of antiretroviral drugs that could select for mutations.

Strain

In the case of HIV, a type of virus, as in "drug-resistant strain."

What matters is not the number, but that we erect a strong barrier against the development of resistance.

28. Should I start treatment?

The answer depends on how you feel, your CD4 count and viral load, and whether you're ready to make the kind of commitment that ART requires. Official guidelines change frequently, but here's what we're thinking now:

1. If you have AIDS, if your CD4 count is less than 200, or if you have serious symptoms caused by HIV, you should start treatment immediately. You're at risk for a large number of serious but preventable complications, some of them fatal.
2. If your CD4 count is between 200 and 500, you should start treatment. You may feel healthy, but your immune system is already been damaged. Why wait for it to get worse?
3. If your CD4 count is over 500, you should consider starting treatment. It's not urgent because your risk of most HIV-related complications is low, but there may other long-term complications that can be prevented by starting ART now, and ART will help you to avoid infecting others. As I write this, two cities, San Francisco and New York, now recommend treatment for all HIV-infected individuals regardless of CD4 count. This is the direction the field is moving in, and may well be what national guidelines will recommend before long.

There are other reasons to start ART regardless of your numbers:

- *Pregnancy.* To prevent transmission to the baby (Question 76).
- *Hepatitis B.* Because you can treat both HIV and hepatitis B with the same drugs (Question 80).

Elite controllers

HIV-infected people whose CD4 counts remain high and whose viral loads remain low without ART.

Antiretroviral drugs work by interfering with one of the stages of the life cycle, and they're classified based on which stage they inhibit.

Drug classes

Categories or groups of HIV drugs that are determined by the way the drugs work and the stage of the viral life cycle that they target.

Entry

The process by which HIV enters human cells. Entry inhibitors are drugs that block entry.

Attachment

The first stage of entry, in which the virus binds to the CD4 receptor.

Entry inhibitors

Drugs that block entry of the virus into the CD4 cell.

* *HIV-associated nephropathy (HIVAN).* Because ART is the only effective treatment (Question 49).
* *Coronary heart disease (or high cardiac risk).* Because HIV increases your risk for heart disease (Question 47).
* *Risk of sexual transmission.* Because lowering your viral load makes you less infectious to others (Question 86).

There are only two groups of people that I advise *not* to start treatment: **elite controllers** (people whose viral loads are un-detectable without treatment), provided they have normal and stable CD4 counts, and those who aren't ready, committed, or capable of adhering to therapy.

29. What are the classes of antiretroviral drugs, and why do they matter?

HIV goes through several stages in its lifespan, beginning with its entry into a human cell and ending with the release of new virus particles into the blood stream that then infect new cells. This is called the viral life cycle (Figure 1). Antiretroviral drugs work by interfering with one of the stages of the life cycle, and they're classified based on which stage they inhibit. Talking about **drug classes** and life cycle stages gets a little technical, but bear with me. Knowing the classes of the drugs isn't essential, but it does help you communicate with your provider. It's also useful because drugs within classes often have overlapping toxicity or resistance patterns. The drugs are listed by category in **Table 3**.

1. **Entry** into the CD4 cell (**entry inhibitors**). This stage has three sub-stages.
   a. **Attachment** of **gp120,** a portion of the **envelope** (the outer part of the virus) to the **CD4 receptor** on the surface of the CD4 cell. There are no **attachment inhibitors** approved yet, but they're being developed.
   b. Binding of coreceptors to gp120. There are two **core-ceptors (or chemokines)** on the cell surface—**CCR5** and **CXCR4.** A drug that blocks CCR5 (**CCR5 antagonist**) is now available (maraviroc or *Selzentry*), and

Table 3 Antiretroviral Agents

Generic Name	Brand Name	Abbreviation	Manufacturer (of brand-name versions)
Nucleoside and nucleotide analog reverse transcriptase inhibitors (NRTIs)			
Abacavir	*Ziagen*	ABC	ViiV Healthcare
Didanosine	*Videx, Videx EC,* or generic	ddI, ddI EC	Bristol-Myers Squibb
Emtricitabine	*Emtriva*	FTC	Gilead Sciences
Lamivudine	*Epivir* or generic	3TC	ViiV Healthcare
Stavudine	*Zerit* or generic	d4T	Bristol-Myers Squibb
Tenofovir disoproxil fumarate	*Viread*	TDF	Gilead Sciences
Zidovudine	*Retrovir* or generic	AZT, ZDV	ViiV Healthcare
Non-nucleoside reverse transcriptase inhibitors (NNRTIs)			
Delavirdine	*Rescriptor*	DLV	ViiV Healthcare
Efavirenz	*Sustiva (Stocrin**)*	EFV	Bristol-Myers Squibb (Merck & Co.**)
Nevirapine	*Viramune* and *Viramune XR*	NVP	Boehringer-Ingelheim
Etravirine	*Intelence*	ETR	Janssen Therapeutics
Rilpivirine	*Edurant*	RPV	Janssen Therapeutics
Protease inhibitors (PIs)			
Atazanavir	*Reyataz*	ATV	Bristol-Myers Squibb
Darunavir	*Prezista*	DRV	Janssen Therapeutics
Fosamprenavir	*Lexiva (Telzir**)*	FPV	ViiV Healthcare
Indinavir	*Crixivan*	IDV	Merck & Co.
Lopinavir/ritonavir	*Kaletra*	LPV/r	Abbott Laboratories
Nelfinavir	*Viracept*	NFV	Pfizer (Roche**)
Ritonavir	*Norvir*	RTV	Abbott Laboratories
Saquinavir	*Invirase*	SQV	Roche
Tipranavir	*Aptivus*	TPV	Boehringer-Ingelheim
Fusion inhibitor			
Enfuvirtide	*Fuzeon*	ENF (T20)	Roche
CCR5 antagonists			
Maraviroc	*Selzentry (Celsentri**)*	MVC	ViiV Healthcare
Integrase inhibitors			
Raltegravir	*Isentress*	RAL	Merck & Co.
Elvitegravir	Not approved*	EVG	Gilead Sciences
Dolutegravir	Not approved*	DTG	ViiV Healthcare
Combination pills			
Abacavir/lamivudine	*Epzicom (Kivexa**)*	ABC/3TC	ViiV Healthcare
Lopinavir/ritonavir	*Kaletra (Aluvia**)*	LPV/r	Abbott Laboratories
Tenofovir/emtricitabine	*Truvada*	TDF/FTC	Gilead Sciences
Tenofovir/emtricitabine/ efavirenz	*Atripla*	TDF/FTC/EFV	Gilead Sciences/Bristol-Myers Squibb
Tenofovir/emtricitabine/ rilpivirine	*Complera (Eviplera**)*	TDF/FTC/RPV	Gilead Sciences
Zidovudine/lamivudine	*Combivir* or generic	AZT/3TC	ViiV Healthcare
Zidovudine/lamivudine/ abacavir	*Trizivir*	AZT/3TC/ABC	ViiV Healthcare
Tenofovir/emtricitabine/ elvitegravir/cobicistat	Not approved*	TDF/FTC/ EVG/COBI	Gilead Sciences

*Drugs not FDA-approved as of 2/1/12.
**Brand names/manufacturers in some countries outside the United States.

gp120

The part of the envelope (outer surface) of HIV that binds to receptors on the surface of the CD4 cell, allowing entry into the cell.

Envelope

The outer surface of the HIV virus.

CD4 receptor

A protein on the surface of the CD4 cell that the virus attaches to before entering the cell.

Coreceptor (or chemokines)

Proteins on the surface of the CD4 cell and other cells that the virus binds to after attaching to the CD4 receptor but before entering the cell.

CCR5 and CXCR4

Coreceptors on the cell surface.

CCR5 antagonist

A drug that blocks CCR5.

Tropism assay

A blood test used to find out whether your virus enters the CD4 cell using the CCR5 coreceptor (R5 virus) or the CXCR4 coreceptor (X4 virus).

others are being developed. We don't have any drugs that block CXCR4 attachment yet. Before using a CCR5 inhibitor, you need a special blood test called a **tropism assay** to make sure you have purely **R5 virus** (virus that enters the cell using only the CCR5 coreceptor). If some of your virus gets in through CXCR4 (**X4** or **dual/mixed [D/M] virus**), it won't be suppressed by the drug.

c. **Fusion** (merging) of the coating of the virus with the surface of the CD4 cell, which allows the genetic material (RNA) of the virus to enter the cell. We now have one approved fusion inhibitor—enfuvirtide (*Fuzeon*).

2. **Reverse transcription** turns viral RNA into DNA. It's called "reverse" because it's the opposite of normal transcription, which turns DNA into RNA. This process requires **reverse transcriptase (RT)**, which is an enzyme (protein) that's brought into the cell from the virus. There are two types of reverse transcriptase inhibitors.

a. **Nucleoside analog reverse transcriptase inhibitors (NRTIs or "nukes")** mimic the normal building blocks of DNA. They get inserted into the growing DNA chain, but because they're not the right nucleosides, they "muck up" the process, stopping the DNA chain from being formed.

b. **Non-nucleoside reverse transcriptase inhibitors (NNRTIs)** stop the same process, but they do it by binding directly to the reverse transcriptase enzyme, preventing it from doing its dirty work.

3. **Integration** is the insertion of the newly created viral DNA into the human DNA in the cell's nucleus. This step requires a viral enzyme called **integrase.** Integrase inhibitors prevent integrase from doing its job.

4. **Protease inhibitors (PIs)** block a late stage in the viral life cycle in which proteins created from viral DNA are cleaved (cut) to create the building blocks of the new viral particles.

Michael's comment:
Whether or not you understand this—I don't, except for a few random words—the good news is that the meds work if you take them the way you're supposed to.

30. How do my provider and I choose my first regimen?

Answering a question like this in a book is tricky because my answer could be out-of-date by the time you read this. Things change fast, as new drugs are developed and new data emerge. The Appendix lists a number of resources that can help keep you up-to-date.

First, make sure you've had a baseline resistance test (Question 24) before choosing your regimen. You don't want to take a drug you're already resistant to. Besides being a waste of time and money, it could put the other drugs in your regimen at risk of resistance.

Your provider needs to know a lot about you to help determine the best regimen. What other medical conditions do you have? What other medications do you take? Are your kidneys and liver in good shape? What's your daily schedule like? Do you eat regular meals? Are you likely to miss doses or stop therapy? If you're a woman who's having sex with men and able to get pregnant, are you using reliable birth control?

There are also questions that you need to ask your provider, nurse, or pharmacist before you start. Do I take my meds with food or without? Does the time of day I take the meds matter? How do I get refills? What if I miss a dose (Question 31)? If I run out of one medication, should I still take the others? What side effects can I expect, and what should I do if I get certain side effects (Question 32)? Don't start therapy until your questions have been answered.

Table 4 lists the advantages and disadvantages of the common initial regimens. Most recommended regimens now include either an NNRTI, or a PI, or an integrase inhibitor. Efavirenz* (*Sustiva*) has been is the favored NNRTI for many years because of its long-term safety and effectiveness in many clinical trials, but rilpivirine (*Edurant, Complera*) and nevirapine (*Viramune*) are alternatives for many people. PIs today are

*With the exception of the coformulated products, I generally refer to drugs by their generic names. For the brand names, abbreviations, and manufacturers of these drugs, see Table 3.

R5 virus

HIV that enters the CD4 cell using the CCR5 coreceptor.

X4 (or dual/mixed [D/M]) virus

HIV that enters the CD4 cell using the CXCR4 coreceptor.

Fusion

The final stage of entry in which the envelope of the virus fuses (merges) with the membrane of the cell, allowing entry of the virus into the cells.

Reverse transcription

The conversion of viral RNA into DNA by reverse transcriptase.

Reverse transcriptase (RT)

An enzyme contained within the HIV virus that can turn viral RNA into DNA so it can be inserted into the DNA of human cells.

Starting Treatment

Table 4: Advantages and Disadvantages of Antiretroviral Drugs Commonly Used for Initial Therapy

Recommended initial regimens all consist of two NRTIs (the "backbone") plus one third agent.

Drug	Forms and Brand Names	Advantages	Disadvantages
Nucleoside (NRTI) "Backbone"			
Tenofovir/ emtricitabine (TDF/FTC)	*Truvada* (also part of *Atripla* and *Complera*)	• The preferred NRTI backbone in current guidelines • 2 single tablet regimens (STRs) available: *Atripla* and *Complera* • Extensively studied • Both drugs active against hepatitis B	• Can cause kidney toxicity (monitor creatinine and urinalysis) • May cause more loss of bone density than other drugs
Abacavir/ lamivudine (ABC/3TC)	*Epzicom* (and part of *Trizivir*)	• Doesn't cause kidney toxicity	• Must pre-test with HLA B*5701 to avoid ABC hypersensitivity reaction (HSR) • Less effective than TDF/FTC in people with viral loads above 100,000 • May increase risk of heart attack (controversial) • No STRs currently available • An alternative NRTI backbone in DHHS Guidelines
Third Agents			
Non-nucleoside reverse transcriptase inhibitors (NNRTIs)			
Efavirenz (EFV)	*Sustiva* (and part of *Atripla*)	• The preferred NNRTI in current guidelines • Extensively studied • STR available (*Atripla*) • Remains in blood for a long time: "forgiving" of missed doses	• Can cause neurologic or psychiatric side effects, especially in the first few weeks • Can cause rash • Resistance common if treatment fails • May cause birth defects if given to pregnant women during the first trimester • Less CD4 increase than with other third agents (PIs, integrase inhibitors)
Rilpivirine (RPV)	*Edurant* (and part of *Complera*)	• STR available (*Complera*) • Better tolerated than *Sustiva, Atripla* (less rash, neurologic side effects, and effect on lipids)	• Less effective than EFV in people with viral loads above 100,000 • Must be taken with a meal • Can't be taken with proton pump inhibitors (PPIs), drugs used to treat reflux and ulcers • Resistance common if treatment fails • Failure may cause cross-resistance to etravirine (*Intelence*) • Classified as an "alternative" NNRTI in current guidelines

Table 4: Advantages and Disadvantages of Antiretroviral Drugs Commonly Used for Initial Therapy

Recommended initial regimens all consist of two NRTIs (the "backbone") plus one third agent.

Drug	Forms and Brand Names	Advantages	Disadvantages
Continued			
Nevirapine (NVP)	*Viramune* and *Viramune XR*	• Well tolerated • Safest NNRTI in pregnancy	• Can cause severe liver toxicity or skin rash during first few weeks, especially in women with pre-treatment CD4 counts above 250 or men with counts above 400 • Resistance common if treatment fails • Classified as an "acceptable" NNRTI in current guidelines
Third Agents **Protease Inhibitors (PIs)**			
Atazanavir/ ritonavir (ATV/r) or atazanavir (ATV)	*Reyataz/ Norvir* or *Reyataz*	• A preferred PI in current guidelines • Lowest number of pills among the PIs • The best PI if ritonavir boosting not possible • Resistance unlikely with failure	• Can cause jaundice • Must be taken with food • Should not be taken with PPIs • Can cause kidney stones (uncommon)
Darunavir/ ritonavir (DRV/r)	*Prezista/ Norvir*	• A preferred PI in current guidelines • Resistance unlikely with failure	• Must be taken with food • Can cause rash
Lopinavir/ ritonavir (LPV/r)	*Kaletra*	• Lopinavir and ritonavir booster included in same pill • Best studied PI in pregnant women • Resistance unlikely with failure	• More GI side effects than ATV or DRV • Affects cholesterol and triglycerides more than ATV or DRV • An altenative PI in current guidelines
Integrase Inhibitors			
Raltegravir (RAL)	*Isentress*	• Few side effects • A preferred agent in current guidelines	• Twice-daily dosing
Elvitegravir (EVG)	Not approved*	• To be approved as part of 4-drug ("quad") STR (with TDF/FTC/cobicistat) • "Quad" as effective as other preferred regimens • No EFV or PI side effects	• Avoid "quad" with abnormal kidney function • More nausea than with some other regimens

*Drug not FDA-approved as of 2/1/12.

Starting Treatment

Nucleoside analog reverse transcriptase inhibitors (NRTIs or "nukes")

A class of antiretroviral drugs that blocks reverse transcription of viral RNA into DNA by mimicking nucleosides, the normal building blocks of DNA.

Non-nucleoside reverse transcriptase inhibitor (NNRTI)

A class of antiretroviral drugs that blocks reverse transcription of viral RNA into DNA by interfering with the activity of reverse transcriptase.

Integration

The insertion of viral DNA into human DNA in the nucleus of the cell.

Integrase

A viral enzyme that allows integration (insertion) of viral DNA into human DNA.

Protease

A viral enzyme that cuts large viral proteins into smaller proteins, which are then used to create new virus particles.

virtually always **boosted** with low doses of ritonavir (*Norvir*) a PI that's too toxic to use at full dose, but lower doses increase drug levels of other PIs, making them stronger and allowing you to take them less often or with fewer pills. Other "boosters" are being studied, and by the time you read this, cobicistat may have been approved for this purpose. The favored PIs for initial therapy are atazanavir (*Reyataz*) and darunavir (*Prezista*), but lopinavir is also widely used, especially in pregnant women. With lopinavir, the ritonavir is already combined (**coformulated**) in the same tablet (*Kaletra*); with the other PIs, the ritonavir is taken separately, though coformulations of PIs with cobicistat are being developed. In addition to the NNRTI, PI, or integrase inhibitor, we typically use a coformulated pill that contains two NRTIs. The usual choices are *Truvada* (tenofovir + emtricitabine) or *Epzicom* (abacavir + lamivudine), though *Combivir* (zidovudine + lamivudine) is still sometimes used and is now available in generic form.

Typical starting regimens are taken once a day with few pills. We now have two single daily tablet regimens, *Atripla*, which contains tenofovir, emtricitabine, and efavirenz and *Complera*, which contains tenofovir, emtricitabine, and rilpivirine. It's expected that a single tablet "quad" coformulation of tenofovir, emtricitabine, elvitegravir, and cobicistat will be approved in 2012, and more coformulated products are being developed. *Atripla* may be more potent than *Complera*, especially for people with high viral loads (above 100,000), but *Complera* is easier to take, since it's less likely to cause neurologic side effects (Question 52) or rash. These convenient regimens aren't appropriate for everyone though. For example, you can't take efavirenz if you were infected with a virus that's resistant to NNRTIs; people with kidney disease shouldn't take tenofovir; efavirenz can cause birth defects in women who get pregnant while taking it; and rilpivirine can't be taken with some medications used to treat ulcers or reflux. Also, if you're not sure you're going to be able to take your pills every day without interruption, you might be better off on a PI, which is less prone to resistance. Raltegravir (*Isentress*) is very effective and well tolerated, though it has to be taken twice a day, unlike the other preferred options. I generally avoid starting with zidovudine (AZT, *Retrovir*, including *Combivir*) or stavudine because of its toxicity, and there's no reason to ever use stavudine (d4T, *Zerit*) anymore (Question 45).

31. Why is adherence so important?

Adherence (or **compliance**) is the word your care provider uses to describe your ability to "stick to" treatment recommendations, especially taking medications. Adherence is important for any medical treatment, but it's *especially* important for HIV infection because of the risk of drug resistance. If you were non-adherent with blood pressure medications, you might damage your heart, kidneys, or vision, but at least the drugs would still work if you started taking them properly. In contrast, HIV is a living organism whose sole purpose in life is to replicate (reproduce itself). ART stops that replication. Missed doses and interruptions in treatment allow drug levels to fall, sometimes low enough to allow the virus to start replicating again. When it does, resistant mutants—virus particles that can replicate in the presence of drugs—will have an advantage. They can eventually replace the non-resistant (wild-type) virus as the dominant viral strain.

For a particularly vivid analogy that you won't soon forget, imagine a can full of your least favorite animals: rats, cockroaches, spiders, or snakes—your choice. If you keep the lid on the can, the critters can't get out. But if you open the lid, the strongest ones will escape, and when they do, they'll hook up with other strong escapees and breed super-creatures that you won't want to have around. ART is the lid on the can. Keep it tightly closed!

Studies show that your ability to adhere to therapy has little to do with your race, sex, education level, or socioeconomic status. Things that *do* affect adherence are mental illness (including depression), drug or alcohol abuse, memory problems,

Boosted protease inhibitors

These combine a protease inhibitor (PI) with a low dose of ritonavir (*Norvir*), another PI that is used only to increase drug levels and prolong the half-life of other PIs.

Coformulated

When two or more drugs are combined into a single tablet or capsule.

Adherence (or compliance)

The term used to refer to a patient's behavior with respect to following treatment recommendations, including taking medications, keeping medical appointments, etc.

Starting Treatment

and a chaotic lifestyle. If any of those issues apply to you, address them before starting therapy (see Part 13). I also find that my patients are more likely to adhere if they understand why they're on treatment, why adherence is important, and if they participated in the decision to start treatment. Finally, it helps to have "self-efficacy:" confidence that you have the ability to affect your future by the actions you take in the present.

Fortunately, adherence is easier now because the available regimens are better tolerated, can be taken just once or twice a day, and include fewer pills. The newer drugs each have alonger **half-life** than the older drugs did, which means they last a long time in the blood. That gives you more "wiggle room" in the timing of doses. But missing doses or interrupting treatment is still risky, especially with NNRTIs and integrase inhibitors, because it only takes a single mutation to get high-level resistance. If you're worried about your ability to adhere to therapy, talk to your provider, nurse, or pharmacist before you start therapy. Many HIV clinics have programs that can help with adherence.

A few tips to help you adhere to your therapy:

1. Get a pill box from the pharmacy—one that has labeled compartments for each day and dose. Put your pills in it each week, even if you're only taking one pill per day. You'll never have to wonder whether you took your pills or not—if they're still in the box, you didn't take them yet.
2. Link your doses to something else you do *every* day—eating a meal, brushing your teeth, or making coffee. If you have a cup of coffee every morning, put your pills beside the coffee maker so you see them when you reach for your morning cup.
3. Always check your medication supply and order your refills in advance—don't run out on weekends or holidays. If you're using a mail-order pharmacy, you have to plan even further ahead.

4. Talk to your provider or pharmacist about what to do if you forget a dose. With most HIV drugs, it's OK to take them as soon as you remember, or even to double the next dose, but I wouldn't suggest doubling the dose of efavirenz because of the side effects you're likely to experience.

My patients who do best are the ones who are a little obsessive-compulsive about taking their medications. When I ask "How many doses have you missed since I saw you last?" they look at me as though I'd asked them about the last time they'd clubbed a group of baby seals.

Michael's comments:
I talk sternly to myself about the importance of taking my medicine as prescribed. My goal is to never miss a dose. I NEVER consult my mood when it's time to take my medicine. There is no good enough reason to miss a dose, and besides, the virus isn't reasonable. The tools I use are a pillbox and good, healthy, empowering fear. The fear reminds me why I need to take meds, and the pillbox tells me whether or not I've taken them. Taking every dose, as prescribed, gives me peace of mind—I'm doing what I need to do to help myself. And it only takes a minute or two a day. I now take my meds once a day (down from three times a day), and I also take medicine for high cholesterol, osteoporosis, and herpes. I've been taking meds for over 10 years now, so I figure I've taken around 10,000 doses. While I never forget that I need to take medication, remembering each dose as a discreet event is impossible. The pillbox is a fail-safe tool.

32. What if I have side effects?

I'll been using two terms—**side effects** and **toxicity**, which are not always the same thing. Side effects make your life unpleasant, but they don't always mean that the drugs are hurting you (for example, nervous system side effects from efavirenz, discussed in Question 52). In contrast, you may feel

Side effects

Undesirable effects of a medication or treatment that are noticeable to the person being treated.

Toxicity

Damage to the body caused by a drug or other substance.

fine even though you're taking a drug that's causing toxicity (for example, high cholesterol from PIs, Question 43). Finally, you may have a side effect that's also a toxicity such as painful feet caused by nerve damage from stavudine (Questions 45 and 52).

Since you'll be starting at least three new medications at once, it's not unusual to experience side effects. Side effects and toxicities of specific drugs are discussed in Part 8. Some side effects, such as the nervous system side effects of efavirenz or upset stomach with zidovudine, are temporary. Others are chronic but manageable, such as loose stools with PIs. Some can be acute and serious, such as **pancreatitis** with didanosine or **hypersensitivity reactions (HSRs)** with abacavir or nevirapine. Other side effects can get worse with continued use (nerve damage with stavudine) or can cause a risk of long-term problems (high cholesterol or blood sugar due to PIs, which increase the risk of heart disease).

Starting therapy is often a trial and error process. You may end up on a different combination than the one you started. Substituting one drug for another because of side effects is fine; it's a much better strategy than stopping completely and starting over later, which can increase the risk of resistance. When starting your first regimen, it's important to know how to contact your provider if you have unexpected side effects or side effects that you can't live with until your next visit.

33. How should my treatment be monitored?

Once you start therapy, it's important to get lab tests done frequently—usually every month or so—during the first few months. The purpose of monitoring is to make sure you're responding to the medications appropriately and not developing toxicity.

The best measure of response to therapy is your viral load. It should decrease at least ten-fold in the first month, which

Pancreatitis

Inflammation of the pancreas.

Hypersensitivity reactions (HSRs)

Reactions, often allergic, to a medication or other substance.

Starting therapy is often a trial and error process. You may end up on a different combination than the one you started. Substituting one drug for another because of side effects is perfectly fine.

means that if it started out at 100,000, it should be below 10,000. Your viral load should then continue to fall until it becomes undetectable using an **ultrasensitive viral load assay** (less than 20 to 75, depending on the test being used), usually within 4 to 6 months. I generally check the viral load every 4 to 6 weeks until it becomes undetectable, then every 3 to 4 months after that. In my patients who have had undetectable viral loads for many years, I monitor them every 6 months.

The CD4 count should also increase on therapy, though the amount of increase is impossible to predict. The CD4 count is usually drawn at the same time as the viral load, though you could monitor it less frequently (every 6–12 months) if you were trying to save money.

We look for drug toxicity with standard blood tests. The complete blood count (CBC) measures the red and white blood cell counts and the platelet count. The only antiretroviral medication that's likely to affect these counts is zidovudine, which can cause **anemia** (low red blood cell count). A comprehensive chemistry panel includes measurements of kidney function, liver health, and blood sugar. A urinalysis may also be included if you're taking medications that can affect the kidneys (tenofovir or indinavir). You should get a fasting lipid panel at least once a year, especially if you're taking medications that affect cholesterol or triglycerides).

34. Can my HIV drugs interact with other medications?

They sure can, which is why you should always carry a list of all of the medicines you're taking, and show that list to other providers who are treating you. The PIs, NNRTIs, and CCR5 antagonist are the drugs most likely to interact with other medications (and with each other). There are few interactions with NRTIs, fusion inhibitors, and raltegravir. Listing all drug interactions here would be impossible, but I'll make a few points about interactions that are especially common and important.

Starting Treatment

Ultrasensitive viral load assay

A viral load test that measures viral load down to a lower limit of 20 to 75 copies/mL.

Anemia

A deficiency of red blood cells, usually diagnosed by a low hemoglobin or hematocrit on a complete blood count.

Carry a list of all of the medicines you're taking, and show that list to other providers who are treating you.

Statins

The common name for HMG CoA reductase inhibitors, drugs that lower cholesterol.

- *Statins.* The levels of the **statins** (drugs that lower cholesterol) can be increased by PIs, causing muscle breakdown and kidney failure. Some, such as simvastatin (*Zocor*) and lovastatin (*Mevacor*), should not be used at all. Others, such as atorvastatin (*Lipitor*), pravastatin (*Pravachol*), and rosuvastatin (*Crestor*), can generally be used at low doses, though pravastatin should be avoided with darunavir (*Prezista*).
- *Birth control pills.* PIs and NNRTIs may lower drug levels, making them less effective, so you may need to use another method of birth control if you're taking one of these drugs.
- *Rifampin.* Rifampin is a drug used to treat TB. It affects the levels of most PIs and NNRTIs. It shouldn't be taken with any PI or NNRTI except efavirenz. If you're using nevirapine or PIs, rifabutin can be used as an alternative.
- *Steroid sprays.* PIs can increase steroid levels with fluticasone, a common ingredient in nasal sprays or inhalers (*Flonase, Advair, Flovent*). Use alternatives if possible. This interaction can also be a problem with steroid injections used to treat joint pain.
- *Narcotics.* Methadone levels are decreased by some NNRTIs and PIs, which can cause withdrawal. Fentanyl levels can be increased, resulting in overdose.
- *Proton pump inhibitors* (PPIs)*. These drugs, which are used to treat acid reflux and ulcers, *should not be used* with atazanavir or rilpivirine because they can lower their absorption. Other drugs that lower stomach acid, such as antacids and H2-blockers** should be used only with careful separation of the doses.
- *Calcium channel blockers****. PIs can increase the levels of these drugs, used to treat high blood pressure, which can increase the risk of side effects.

*PPIs: Omeprazole (*Prilosec*), esomeprazole (*Nexium*), pantoprazole (*Protonix*), lansoprazole (*Prevacid*), and rabeprazole (*Aciphex*).

**H2-blockers: Ranitidine (*Zantac*), cimetidine (*Tagamet*), and famotidine (*Pepcid*).

***Calcium channel blockers: Nifedipine (*Adalat, Procardia*), verapamil (*Calan*), and diltiazem (*Cardizem, Tiazac,* and others).

- *Seizure medications.* It's important to check drug levels of a number of seizure medications if you're on ART to make sure you're getting the right dose. Some seizure medications can lower drug levels of some HIV drugs.
- *Alternative therapies.* Don't forget that many **complementary medicine** and **alternative medicine** therapies, such as herbal supplements, are *drugs* from the body's point of view and can interact with prescribed medications (Questions 41 and 91).

This is *not* a complete list. When in doubt, ask your provider or pharmacist.

Complementary medicine

The use of a non-standard medical treatment in addition to standard therapy.

Alternative medicine

The use of a non-standard medical treatment in place of standard therapy.

Starting Treatment

PART SEVEN

Staying On Therapy

How long will therapy last?

Can therapy ever be stopped?

How will I know if my treatment stops working?

More . . .

35. How long will therapy last?

If you're taking well-chosen therapy and you're not missing doses, your first regimen can probably last as long as you do, or until something better comes along. In the bad old days, we'd start treatment with zidovudine, would see a rise in CD4 count that might last for a year or two if we were lucky, and then we'd be back where we were before. Then we'd try another NRTI or a combination of two NRTIs, and the benefit would be even shorter. Since we weren't able to fully suppress the viral load with NRTIs, resistance began evolving from the moment they were started. The inevitable result of therapy was resistance to the drug that was being taken and **cross-resistance** to other drugs in the same class.

Things changed completely in the mid-90s with the availability of PIs, NNRTIs, and the concept of combination therapy, not just because we started using three drugs, but because we went from merely decreasing viral replication to stopping it altogether. Now that we can keep the virus from replicating, we can stop mutation from occurring and prevent resistance. It's theoretically possible for the benefits of a single ART regimen to be permanent as long as you continue to take it faithfully.

Some researchers believe that the virus is replicating at very low levels, even when the viral load is undetectable. If they're right, then resistance could emerge eventually, though it might take decades. Others believe that there is no replication and point to studies showing that the virus of highly adherent patients after many years on ART is identical to the one they started, with no evolution of resistance.

My patients aren't failing therapy without a reason. Those who fail are either missing doses of their medications or had a lot of resistance to begin with. When failure does occur, we have plenty of good treatment options. I'm confident that if taken correctly, ART can last for a lifetime.

Cross-resistance

Resistance to one drug that results in resistance to other drugs, usually in the same class.

It's theoretically possible for the benefits of a single ART regimen to be permanent as long as you continue to take it faithfully.

36. Can therapy ever be stopped?

It can, but it's almost always a bad idea. You should assume that once you start therapy, you're in it for the long haul. We used to hear a lot about **treatment interruption** (a **drug holidays** or **structured treatment interruptions**). Patients were tired of side effects and wanted a break. Researchers thought that occasional structured treatment interruptions might allow people to take a break from side effects and recover from drug toxicity without doing harm, provided the CD4 count stayed in a safe zone.

That approach turned out to be very wrong. A large clinical trial comparing intermittent versus continuous therapy was stopped early because people who interrupted therapy were more likely to die or have serious complications than those who remained on therapy, even if they kept their CD4 counts above 250. In short, the concept of treatment interruption as a deliberate strategy is dead in the water.

That doesn't mean you can't stop treatment if you have to. We sometimes have to stop therapy in people who develop serious side effects or who are too sick to take medications, but those are exceptional cases. Fortunately, now that ART has improved, staying on therapy is easier than it used to be. Be aware that stopping NNRTI-containing regimens can be especially risky. The long half-life of drugs like efavirenz, rilpivirine, and nevirapine means that the drugs hang around for a long time—sometimes weeks after your last dose. That's a problem, since resistance to these drugs requires just a single mutation. If you should ever have to stop taking one of these regimens, talk to your provider about safer ways to do it.

37. How will I know if my treatment stops working?

You can't tell whether therapy is working based on how you feel. The only way to know for sure is by measuring the

You should assume that once you start therapy, you're in it for the long haul.

Treatment interruption

Stopping antiretroviral therapy.

Drug holiday

The term for an interruption in therapy when the decision has been made by the patient.

Structured treatment interruption

The term for an interruption in therapy that's been approved by the provider.

Staying On Therapy

viral load: the best measure of treatment success and failure (Question 23). Your viral load should be undetectable using an ultrasensitive viral load assay within 4 to 6 months of starting therapy. If your viral load doesn't decrease the way it's supposed to, or if it becomes detectable after having been undetectable, this *may* be a sign of treatment failure.

No lab test is perfect, however. A viral load can be detectable in people who aren't failing, often just because no lab test is 100 percent accurate. If you're taking your medications faithfully and you have a viral load that's detectable but low, don't panic. It's probably just a "blip"— a single detectable viral load that generally means nothing (Question 23). The only way to tell the difference between a blip and early failure is to repeat the viral load. If it's back to undetectable levels, then it was a blip, and you should forget about it. We generally get concerned only if the viral load is repeatedly above 200.

If the viral load remains detectable or is rising, there may be a problem. This should be taken seriously—even when everything else is going great—because it could mean that you're developing resistance. We can measure resistance when the viral load is above 500 to 1,000 (Question 24).

The CD4 count is a poor measure of treatment failure (Question 22). If your viral load is undetectable but your CD4 response is disappointing, changing medications probably won't make much difference. The best approach is to keep your viral load undetectable, and let the CD4 count do what it will do.

38. What if my virus becomes resistant to the medications?

Resistance can be the *result* of treatment failure (when you're not taking your medications properly) or it can be the *cause* of failure (when you already have resistance before you start). Resistance can occur whenever the virus is able to replicate despite the use of antiretroviral medications. Fortunately, resistance is no longer the inevitable result of treatment, as it was in the pre- HAART era. Studies show that people who take their medications faithfully rarely develop resistance.

The best way to deal with resistance is not to let it happen in the first place. If you're about to start therapy for the first time, get a resistance test to make sure your virus is susceptible. Once you start, take every dose and keep your viral load suppressed. If you follow those two rules, you'll probably never have to read the rest of this answer.

But, to paraphrase an oft-repeated maxim, "resistance happens." When it does, I've got two more rules to live by: (1) Act fast. Continuing a failing regimen allows more mutations and resistance to occur. (2) Get data. Resistance testing tells you which drugs your virus is resistant to and which will still work (Question 24).

We've now got a lot of drugs in different classes and with different resistance profiles. If you develop resistance on your first combination, you'll still have plenty of good treatment options. But those options might not be as easy or as well-tolerated as the first, so make the first one work!

39. Are new drugs being developed?

Since the approval of zidovudine in 1987, there has been a steady increase in the number of new antiretroviral agents. The first drugs were NRTIs. Two other classes, PIs and NNRTIs, were first introduced in the mid-90s. Then came enfuvirtide, a fusion inhibitor and the first entry inhibitor. 2007 was an important year, with the introduction of maraviroc—the first CCR5 antagonist; raltegravir—the first integrase inhibitor; and etravirine—a new "second generation" NNRTI (Question 29). 2011 saw the approval of rilpivirine, a new NNRTI, as well as *Complera*, a single-tablet regimen that contains rilpivirine, tenofovir, and emtricitabine. In 2012 we expect approval of a "quad" pill containing the integrase inhibitor, elvitegravir, the non-ritonavir

Studies show that people who take their medications faithfully rarely develop resistance.

The best way to deal with resistance is not to let it happen in the first place.

Staying On Therapy

booster, cobicistat, tenofovir and emtricitabine, and a third integrase inhibitor, dolutegravir, is also on the way. There are additional entry inhibitors, NRTIs, NNRTIs, and integrase inhibitors being developed.

It costs a lot of money to develop a new drug and to get it approved by the FDA. For a drug to make it that far, it has to have a reason to exist. New drugs tend to fall into one of two categories. They either work when others don't—because of a unique mechanism of action or resistance profile—or they're more convenient or less toxic than similar drugs. In addition, clinical studies must show that the drug is well-absorbed, achieves adequate drug levels, suppresses viral load, and is active and safe. A lot of things can go wrong along the way, and not all drug candidates make it to the finish line.

At some point, drug companies may decide that the current therapies for HIV infection are good enough, and that there's no longer a financial incentive to develop new ones. That hasn't happened yet, but the pace of drug development has definitely slowed, especially for drugs used to treat resistant virus. Don't assume there will always be new drugs to bail you out if you fail multiple regimens. Make your current regimen last by taking it as prescribed.

40. What if I decide not to take medications?

Most HIV-positive people will need treatment at some point. I sometimes hear people say they want to fight their HIV the "natural way" rather than by treating themselves with "toxic chemicals." People who talk like that are usually too young to remember the devastation that AIDS caused during the pre-HAART years, and they're unaware of the devastation that it's still causing in parts of the world that can't afford effective therapy. They also forget that "natural" doesn't always mean healthy. After all, HIV is completely "natural," and it's killing millions. In contrast, those "toxic chemicals" that we doctors like to dish out have saved countless lives and represent one of the great medical miracles of the 20th century.

Although almost everyone with HIV infection could probably benefit from ART, not everyone *needs* to be on therapy. Question 28 talks about who needs to be treated. People with high CD4 counts and low or undetectable viral loads could choose to be monitored without medications. Some people are elite controllers—they have normal CD4 counts, low viral loads, and don't progress despite years of untreated infection. However, they represent a small fraction of HIV-positive people, and they're the way they are because of their own genetic make-up, not because of their lifestyle, diet, herbal supplements, or anything else they have control over.

The AIDS epidemic is over 30 years old now, and we know more than we care to know about the slow, miserable death that results from untreated HIV infection. Why go back to the '80s when you live in the 21st century? Take advantage of what medical science has to offer, and save your life!

41. Should I take complementary or alternative therapies?

Complementary and alternative medicine (CAM) is the term used to describe non-standard therapies. Complementary medicine is the use of non-standard therapy *in addition to* standard therapy; alternative medicine is the use of non-standard therapy *instead of* standard therapy. One problem with non-standard therapies is that there usually isn't enough evidence to make them standard. That doesn't necessarily mean they don't work. Natural therapies can become standard. For example, fish oil is now being used to treat high cholesterol and triglycerides. There are also examples of natural substances that are very bad for you. (Socrates didn't take hemlock for his health!)

Research into the safety and benefits of CAM *is* being conducted. In fact, the National Center for Complementary and Alternative Medicine, which is part of the **National Institutes of Health (NIH),** now gives grants for this kind of research. In some cases, the research supports the claims made

Complementary and alternative medicine (CAM)

Medical products or treatments that are not standard of care.

National Institutes of Health (NIH)

An agency of the federal government (under the Department of Health and Human Services) responsible for conducting and funding medical research.

about these substances; in other cases it doesn't. So far, there have been no alternative therapies for HIV infection that have come close to matching the benefits of ART.

Another problem with CAM is that it often involves taking substances that can interact with ART drugs. Those who think of herbs as cuddly, benign, natural substances don't like to use hear them called "drugs," but let's face it—if they weren't drugs, there would be no point in taking them. Antiretroviral medications interact with lots of other drugs, and we now know they can interact with herbal medications, too. The best studied example is St. John's wort, which lowers PI levels, allowing the virus to replicate and develop resistance. Unfortunately, few of the many CAM therapies have been tested for interactions with HIV drugs.

My advice is to follow the data. Don't be like my patient who was skeptical about all the treatments I suggested but who bought and swallowed everything recommended by the high school drop-out at the local health food store. Be skeptical about *everything*. Whether you're thinking of taking a prescription drug or an herb—first ask, "What's the scientific evidence that this will help me and not hurt me?"

42. What is immune-based therapy?

Immune-based therapy is treatment designed to restore the immune system or to improve its ability to fight HIV infection. It's clear now that we're not going to cure HIV infection just by keeping the viral load undetectable with ART. The virus inserts its DNA into human cells, where it remains forever, waiting until treatment is stopped to create new virus particles. Our drugs only work on replicating virus; they have no activity against viral DNA that's hiding out in resting CD4 cells.

Immune-based therapy

Treatment for HIV infection designed to affect the immune system and its response to the virus, as opposed to standard antiretroviral therapy, which suppresses the virus itself.

Theoretically, we could cure HIV infection if we could activate all resting CD4 cells and wake up the sleeping (latent) virus, which ART could then attack. This has been attempted with drugs like interleukin-2 and with valproic acid. There are two problems with this approach. First, unless you activate *every* resting CD4 cell in the body, you'll still have latent virus, no closer to a cure than you were before. Second, resting CD4 cells aren't the only reservoirs for latent HIV, but the proposed treatments may wake up only CD4 cells.

Another immune-based approach is therapeutic vaccination. The idea here is not to eradicate HIV, but to stimulate the immune system to fight it better. A successful **therapeutic vaccine** might delay the need for ART, turning more people into elite controllers. There are promising vaccines being studied, but this is still an experimental approach that probably won't be put into practice any time soon.

Immune-based therapy has clearly lagged behind antiviral therapy, but that doesn't mean it doesn't have a future. Maybe I'll have better news in the next edition of this book.

Therapeutic vaccine

A vaccine given to treat an existing infection by stimulating the immune system to fight it.

Staying On Therapy

PART EIGHT

Side Effects and Toxicity

What are the side effects of protease inhibitors?

What can I do about body shape changes?

How can I protect my liver?

More . . .

43. What are the side effects of protease inhibitors?

Some side effects and long-term toxicities have been attributed to PIs as a class. These include **gastrointestinal** symptoms, such as loose stools or nausea (Question 66), body shape changes (fat accumulation), and metabolic toxicities, such as increased levels of **cholesterol** and **triglycerides** and high blood sugar or **diabetes**. However, the preferred PIs, atazanavir (*Reyataz*) and darunavir (*Prezista*), are well tolerated and are much less likely to cause these problems than the older PIs.

Hyperlipidemia is an elevation of the cholesterol and/or triglyceride levels. High cholesterol can increase the risk for heart disease and stroke (Question 47). Very high triglyceride levels can cause pancreatitis. If you have high lipids, the first step is to change your diet, perhaps with the help of a nutritionist, and to do more aerobic exercise. Depending on how bad the results are and the number of other cardiac risk factors you have, hyperlipidemia may need to be treated either with medications that lower cholesterol and/or triglycerides or by changing your HIV drugs.

Insulin resistance means the body can't respond appropriately to the insulin that is produced by the **pancreas** to control blood sugar. When it's severe enough, it can lead to diabetes. Some PIs can cause insulin resistance—the best example is indinavir (*Crixivan*). It's detected with a fasting blood sugar test or a glucose tolerance test. People with insulin resistance or diabetes need to change their diet by avoiding sugars, limiting starches, and eating small amounts throughout the day. Aerobic exercise and weight loss helps a lot. Sometimes, this requires treatment with "insulin sensitizing" drugs or a change in your HIV medications. The problem can sometimes get better or go away completely when you stop the drugs that cause it.

Gastrointestinal

Relating to the GI tract: esophagus, stomach, small intestines, colon, and rectum.

Cholesterol

A substance found in body tissues and the blood.

Triglycerides

Fats that are ingested in the form of vegetable oils and animal fats.

Diabetes

A disorder resulting in elevated amounts of glucose (sugar) in the blood and urine.

Hyperlipidemia

An abnormal elevation of lipids (cholesterol and/or triglycerides) in the blood.

Insulin resistance

A condition in which the body cannot respond to insulin as well as it should.

Pancreas

An organ in the abdomen that makes insulin and enzymes that help digest food.

Fat accumulation (or lipohypertrophy) is the build-up of fat in places where it doesn't belong and is discussed further in Question 46.

Liver toxicity (hepatotoxicity) can occur with any PI, but people who have chronic hepatitis B or C are at greatest risk (Question 48). Liver toxicity is something that usually shows up in your blood test results before you feel it yourself. Notify your provider if you develop belly pain, continued nausea, dark urine, or yellow skin or eyes.

Other PI side effects include elevation of **bilirubin** (indinavir or atazanavir), which is completely harmless but may cause jaundice (yellowing of the eyes or skin); kidney stones or kidney damage (indinavir, atazanavir); dry skin, hair loss, cracked lips, and ingrown toenails (indinavir); and rash (fosamprenavir [*Lexiva*] or darunavir).

> *Rose's comment:*
> *The side effects of the protease inhibitors for me are worse during my menstrual cycle. I get diarrhea, abdominal cramps, muscle and joint aches, and gas pain. I know it's the protease inhibitor because I didn't take it for 2 days and the side effects went away. (Joel wasn't happy with me for stopping my meds!!)*
>
> *Back when I was using drugs like AZT and d4T, my legs got skinny, and I gained weight in my belly. Weight gain is still a problem, though Joel tells me I can't blame it all on the drugs. He claims I should diet and exercise, but what does he know?*
>
> *Over the years, I've had plenty of other side effects that aren't worth mentioning because they happened with old drugs, and things are a lot better now. But not taking them has never been a question. The side effects have been a small price to pay for my life!*

Side Effects and Toxicity

Fat accumulation (or lipohypertrophy)
A component of the "lipodystrophy syndrome" in which fat accumulates in abnormal parts of the body, such as inside the abdomen, around the neck, in the breasts, or on the upper back at the base of the neck ("buffalo hump").

Liver toxicity (hepatotoxicity)
Damage to the liver caused by medications.

Bilirubin
A pigment produced in the liver.

44. What are the side effects of non-nucleoside reverse transcriptase inhibitors (NNRTIs)?

NNRTIs have little long-term toxicity, but they do have some short-term side effects you should know about.

- *Rash.* All of the NNRTIs can cause a rash, usually during the first few weeks of therapy. It's an itchy, red rash, which usually gets better on its own even if you continue the drug. However, severe, even life-threatening rashes can occur, especially with nevirapine (*Viramune*). Signs of a serious rash are peeling or blistering of the skin, sores in the mouth, or fever. Nevirapine is given once a day for the first 2 weeks, then twice a day, but never increase the dose if you've got a rash. Rash can occur with efavirenz (*Sustiva, Atripla*), but it's less likely to be severe or to require stopping the drug. Rilpivirine (*Edurant, Complera*) causes less rash than either nevirapine or efavirenz.
- *Liver toxicity.* Nevirapine can cause serious, acute liver toxicity during the first few weeks of therapy, especially in women who start the drug with CD4 counts above 250 or men with counts over 400. Always see your provider and get your liver labs checked before you increase the dose of nevirapine after the first 2 weeks. People with chronic hepatitis B or C can take nevirapine, but they are at higher risk for chronic liver toxicity and should be monitored carefully.
- *Hyperlipidemia.* NNRTIs can elevate cholesterol and/or triglycerides but usually to a lesser degree than with most of the PIs. Efavirenz has a bigger effect on lipids than nevirapine or rilpivirine.
- *Neurologic side effects.* Efavirenz often causes vivid dreams (good or bad), dizziness, and concentration difficulties during the first few days or weeks of treatment. Tips on managing these side effects are discussed in Question 52.

45. What should I know about nucleoside analog side effects?

- *Neuropathy (or peripheral neuropathy).* Stavudine (d4T, *Zerit*) and didanosine (ddI, *Videx*), which are no longer widely used, can cause **neuropathy**: damage to the nerves in your feet and legs. The first symptoms are tingling, numbness, or burning pain in the toes. With time, this can extend up into the legs and become disabling. If you change drugs when the symptoms are limited to the toes, the neuropathy should go away quickly.

- *Lactic acidosis and hepatic steatosis.* **Lactic acidosis** and **hepatic steatosis** are are uncommon but serious side effects, mainly of stavudine, but to a lesser degree of zidovudine (AZT, *Retrovir, Combivir, Trizivir*) and possibly didanosine. Symptoms can include shortness of breath, nausea, muscle aches, and just feeling lousy. Of course, these are common symptoms, while lactic acidosis isn't common at all. If you're having them, it doesn't mean you have lactic acidosis, but you should report them to your provider. Early diagnosis and a change in therapy are essential, since lactic acidosis can be fatal.

- *Lipoatrophy.* Fat loss in the face, arms, legs, and buttocks (discussed in Question 46) can be caused by stavudine and to a lesser degree by zidovudine and possibly didanosine.

- *Anemia.* Zidovudine can cause anemia. Symptoms include fatigue, dizziness, and shortness of breath. A standard blood test (CBC) will detect anemia.

- *Gastrointestinal side effects.* Zidovudine can cause nausea; tenofovir (TDF, *Viread, Atripla, Complera*) can cause gas or bloating. NRTIs generally don't cause diarrhea. Didanosine can cause pancreatitis, a dangerous inflammation of the pancreas. Get medical attention immediately if you're taking didanosine and you develop bad belly pain.

Neuropathy (or peripheral neuropathy)
Damage to the nerves resulting in numbness or burning pain, usually in the feet or legs.

Lactic acidosis
A dangerous build-up of lactic acid (lactate) in the blood, which can be caused by some antiretroviral drugs and also by other medical conditions.

Hepatic steatosis
A build-up of fat in the liver that can be caused by a variety of medical conditions.

Side Effects and Toxicity

- *Hypersensitivity.* People taking abacavir (*Ziagen*, *Epzicom*, *Trizivir*, *Kivexa*) can develop a hypersensitivity reaction (HSR) within the first few weeks. HSR feels like the flu and gets worse with each dose. If you think you're having HSR, talk to your provider immediately because it's important to be sure. Once you stop abacavir because of possible HSR, you can never take it again because there have been deaths in people who were "rechallenged" with abacavir after having had HSR. Caucasians are at greatest risk. However, the risk of HSR has been virtually eliminted by pre-testing for HLA B*5701. Get the test before taking abacavir, and if it's positive don't take abacavir in any of its forms. If you're negative, you're *very* unlikely to get HSR.
- *Kidney problems.* Tenofovir can affect the kidneys, usually in people who already have kidney problems to begin with. The risk is higher if you're also taking a protease inhibitor. Kidney problems will be detected by standard blood and urine tests.
- *Metabolic toxicity.* Lipid elevation and insulin resistance usually get blamed on protease inhibitors, but NRTIs can cause them, too, especially stavudine and zidovudine.

46. What can I do about body shape changes?

Lipodystrophy

A general term for changes in body shape and fat distribution caused by some antiretroviral agents.

Lipoatrophy

Loss of subcutaneous fat (fat under the skin) in the legs, arms, buttocks, and face, caused by some nucleoside analog reverse transcriptase inhibitors (NRTIs).

Lipodystrophy is a term used to describe body shape changes that can occur with antiretroviral therapy. Lipodystrophy includes **lipoatrophy** (fat loss) and fat accumulation. You can have one or the other or—bad luck!—you can have both. Fortunately, these are no longer common problems because of the greater safety of the drugs we use today.

Lipoatrophy

Loss of fat in the arms, legs, and buttocks makes your veins stand out and gives you a flat or saggy butt. Loss of fat in the face gives you sunken cheeks and makes you look older or sicker than you are. Stavudine (d4T, *Zerit*) and zidovudine

(AZT, *Retrovir, Combivir, Trizivir*) are the most common causes of lipotrophy, but didanosine (ddI, *Videx*) may cause it too. The best way to deal with lipoatrophy is to avoid the drugs that cause it. If you're on one of those drugs and you notice changes in your appearance, switch drugs before it gets worse. Some fat will come back, but it can take a long time if you've lost a lot, and we still don't know whether things ever return to normal. There are cosmetic procedures that treat lipoatrophy in the face, such as the use of "face filler" injections like polylactic acid (*Sculptra*).

Fat Accumulation

Fat can appear in unusual places, such as the upper back ("buffalo hump"), around the neck, in the breast tissue, or inside the abdomen. As a general rule, belly fat that you can grab between your fingers is **subcutaneous fat** (fat under the skin), which is normal and can't be blamed on your drugs. Abnormal fat is **visceral fat** (fat inside the belly), which can make your stomach stick out but can't be pinched.

The cause of fat accumulation is not completely clear. It's been linked to PIs, possibly because of their tendency to increase triglycerides and cause insulin resistance (Question 43). Sometimes fat gain isn't really a side effect of medications at all but is the result of improved overall health due to antiretroviral therapy. To put it simply, now that you're feeding yourself instead of the virus, you're "catching up"—gaining the weight you *would* have had if you didn't have HIV infection.

If you're developing fat accumulation, make sure you get checked for hyperlipidemia and insulin resistance, and deal with those problems if you have them. Then, get off the couch, replace the potato chips with carrot sticks, and get to the gym. Diet and exercise will help, whether you've got fat accumulation or just plain fat. For true fat visceral accumulation, there are treatments that can help, including growth

Subcutaneous fat

Fat found under the skin.

Visceral fat

Fat present inside the abdomen, around the internal organs, rather than under the skin.

hormone (*Serostim*) and tesamoralin (*Egrifta*). However, these are expensive drugs, and the fat tends to return after you stop taking them.

Michael's comment:
I complained to Dr. Gallant about my belly for a couple years. Each time he'd ask me about my diet and exercise routine. I'd tell him that I couldn't change either. Anyway, I'd decided that the fat was visceral (the kind you can't grab), caused by meds, and that it was my fate to be fat. A couple months ago my boyfriend decided to lose weight, and I joined him, partly so I wouldn't be rubbing my hollandaise into his face. Lo and behold, eating fewer calories and spending extra time at the gym every day adds up to a lower number on the bathroom scale. I don't know that I'll ever achieve the flat, tomboy stomach of my dreams (what's your opinion, Dr. Gallant?), but working toward a goal seems more productive that sitting on the sofa with a tub of Rocky Road, grousing.

47. Am I at higher risk for heart disease?

Studies have shown that HIV-positive people are at higher risk for heart disease and heart attack than the general population. However, the increased risk is partly due to the effects of HIV itself, and is reduced with ART. Some antiretroviral drugs can increase the risk of heart disease. For example, some PIs and NRTIs can cause elevations in cholesterol, insulin resistance, and fat accumulation (Questions 43, 45, and 46), all of which are risk factors for heart disease. There is an ongoing controversy about whether abacavir (*Ziagen*, *Epzicom*, *Trizivir*) increases the risk of heart attack.

It's important to put the increased risk in context. First, your risk of a heart attack if you take ART is tiny in comparison to your risk of dying of AIDS if you don't. Second, the risk from ART may be small in comparison to the effects of other risk factors that you have control over, such as high cholesterol, insulin resistance and diabetes, high blood pressure, smoking, obesity, and inactivity. Finally, you lower your cardiac risk by treating HIV far more than you increase it by taking ART.

Here's how to protect your heart: (1) don't smoke, (2) quit smoking (3) don't even think about lighting up that cigarette (4) get your blood pressure under control if it's high, (5) get your cholesterol down if it's high, (6) keep your blood sugar in control if you've got diabetes, and (7) keep your weight down with aerobic exercise and a healthy diet. That leaves only three other risk factors—getting older, being a man (if you are one), and bad genes—and you can't do anything about them.

…Oh, and did I mention that you shouldn't smoke?

48. How can I protect my liver?

The liver is a vitally important organ, though many people are unclear about what it actually does. Its functions are too numerous to list completely, but it's involved in metabolism, the chemical reactions that take place in the cells of the body, including the **detoxification** of many of the drugs we use to treat HIV. It makes proteins, stores fuel for the body, and secretes important hormones and bile, which helps with digestion of food. Since it's so important, it's a good idea to keep it healthy.

Detoxification

The removal of toxic substances from the body.

Many antiretroviral drugs can hurt the liver. Almost all of the PIs can cause damage, but usually only in people who have chronic hepatitis B or C. Nevirapine (*Viramune*) can be harmful to the liver, especially in women with high CD4 counts. Stavudine (d4T, *Zerit*) and zidovudine (AZT, *Retrovir, Combivir, Trizivir*) can be harmful, too, especially if you also have lactic acidosis. Other medications commonly taken by HIV-positive people, such as cholesterol-lowering drugs, can also cause liver toxicity. Here are some tips for lowering your risk.

1. Get checked for hepatitis A, B, and C. If you're not already immune to A and B, get vaccinated (preferably after you've started ART). If you have chronic hepatitis B or C, get evaluated by an expert to find out whether you need treatment (Questions 79 and 80). PCR tests are sometimes necessary to rule out hepatitis since it's possible to have hepatitis with negative serologies.

2. Get your **transaminases (liver enzymes)** checked frequently, especially when you've just started therapy. This is especially important with nevirapine (Question 44).

3. Avoid excessive alcohol use (Question 92). Don't drink at all if you have chronic hepatitis B or C.

4. Use acetaminophen, the active ingredient in *Tylenol* and many other over-the-counter remedies, in moderation, and not at all if you have chronic hepatitis.

5. If you're taking medications for hepatitis B, don't stop them. Stopping treatment can cause dangerous hepatitis flares.

There are some who recommend herbal therapies, especially milk thistle, to "detoxify" or protect the liver, though the data are mixed. Some "natural products" may actually hurt the liver and worsen liver disease. There's no clear evidence that there's anything you can take to protect the liver.

49. Should I worry about my kidneys?

The kidneys are organs that filter your blood and get rid of some of the things you don't need. There are only a few things you need to know about the kidneys from an HIV standpoint.

- *HIV-associated nephropathy (HIVAN).* Black people get the raw end of the deal when it comes to kidney problems. They're at greater risk for kidney failure due to diabetes, hypertension, and also HIV infection. Among HIV-positive blacks **HIVAN** is a fairly common cause of kidney failure requiring dialysis or transplantation. The first clue is that there's protein in the urine. The diagnosis

---

Transaminases (liver enzymes)

Blood tests used to look for damage to the liver.

The kidneys are organs that filter your blood and get rid of some of the things you don't need.

Nephropathy, HIV-associated (HIVAN)

A disease of the kidneys caused by HIV infection.

is usually made by removing a small piece of the kidney with a needle (**kidney biopsy**). If you've got HIVAN, you should start ART right away, since it's the only truly effective treatment.

- *Drug toxicity.* Indinavir (*Crixivan*), now rarely used, can cause kidney stones and can damage kidney function, which is one of the reasons we don't use it much anymore. Tenofovir (*Viread, Atripla, Complera*) can also hurt the kidneys, but usually in people who already have kidney problems. If your kidneys aren't working well, then tenofovir may not be the best drug for you. Atazanavir (*Reyataz*) can sometimes cause kidney stones.

- Be careful with other drugs that hurt the kidneys, such as **non-steroidal anti-inflammatory drugs (NSAIDs)** (ibuprofen, naproxen, and related drugs, which are found in many over-the-counter medications, such as *Motrin* and *Aleve*). Many of the other NRTIs should be given at reduced doses if you have kidney problems, even though they don't directly affect the kidneys themselves. HIV-positive people often take other drugs that can cause kidney problems, including **trimethoprim-sulfamethoxazole** (TMP-SMX, cotrimoxazole, *Bactrim, Septra*).

Kidney problems are detected with standard monitoring tests—the serum creatinine included in the comprehensive chemistry panel and a urinalysis.

50. Are there risks to my bones and joints?

Bone and joint problems are now being recognized as a complication of HIV infection, HIV therapy, or both. There are two distinct problems—osteopenia/osteoporosis and osteonecrosis.

- **Osteopenia** is loss of bone density. When it becomes severe enough, it can result in **osteoporosis** (severe thinning of the bones leading to fractures). You lose some bone density after you start ART, and probably more when the

kidney biopsy

A procedure in which a piece of a kidney is removed using a needle inserted through the skin in order to find out the cause of kidney disorders.

Non-steroidal anti-inflammatory drugs (NSAIDs)

Drugs that are commonly used to suppress inflammation and treat pain.

Trimethoprim-sulfamethoxazole (TMP-SMX, cotrimoxazole, Bactrim, Septra)

An antibiotic used to treat or prevent PCP and to prevent toxoplasmosis.

Osteopenia

A loss of bone density ("thinning of the bones").

Osteoporosis

Severe osteopenia, which can lead to bone fractures.

Side Effects and Toxicity

regimen contains tenofovir (*Viread, Atripla, Complera*), but the amount is small, and bone density generally levels off quickly without progressing further. However, HIV infection probably causes bone loss too, and there's some evidence that people who have ever had low CD4 counts are at greater risk for bone fractures. Other risk factors for osteopenia include smoking, use of corticosteroids (prednisone), low testosterone levels (hypogonadism, Question 51), older age, and lower CD4 count. Vitamin D deficiency, a common condition in people with HIV and in the general population, is another risk factor for loss of bone density, and may be more common or more severe in people taking efavirenz (*Sustiva, Atripla*). The diagnosis of ostepenia or osteoporosis is made by DEXA scan, which is now recomended as a routine test in HIV-positive men over 50 and post-menopausal women. Taking vitamin D supplements, getting adequate calcium in the diet, and resistance (muscle-building) exercise can also help preserve bone density. ART probably helps, too.

Osteonecrosis

Damage to bones at the large joints.

Avascular necrosis

Painful joint damage caused by osteo-necrosis, usually affecting the hips but sometimes the shoulders.

- **Osteonecrosis** is the underlying cause of **avascular necrosis,** a destruction of large joints, usually the hips. We don't know what causes it; we only know that it's more common in HIV-positive people. The most common symptom is hip pain. Standard x-rays may not detect it; you usually need an MRI of the hips to make the diagnosis. The only treatment is surgical—usually hip replacement.

We still have a lot to learn about bone and joint problems. We need to know whether they're caused by ART in general, specific drugs, or just by living a long time with HIV infection. Does ART prevent bone problems , or cause them? I hope to have more answers for you in the next edition.

51. Can HIV or ART affect my hormones?

They can. Here are some examples:

- *Hypogonadism.* HIV-positive men sometimes have low testosterone levels (**hypogonadism**); we see it in men with advanced HIV disease, where it's assumed to be a result of being sick, but also in healthy men on effective ART, where it *may* be a side effect of medications. Symptoms include fatigue, loss of sex drive or performance, weight loss, muscle wasting, or the inability to gain weight. The diagnosis is made with a morning blood **testosterone** level (the free level is usually more accurate than the total). The condition is treated with testosterone gels, patches, or injections. Testosterone should only be used in men with low testosterone levels. If your levels are normal, taking testosterone will make your testicles lazy. They'll see no reason to keep producing testosterone themselves, and they'll shrivel up into little hazelnuts. If you didn't have hypogonadism before, you'll have it now.
- *Insulin resistance and diabetes.* See Question 43.
- *Thyroid disease.* Thyroid problems aren't much more common in HIV-positive people than in anyone else, but if there's any question about whether you have thyroid problems, it's easy enough to check using a test called TSH.
- *Adrenal problems.* **Adrenal insufficiency** (low levels of **cortisol**, a hormone produced by the **adrenal glands**) isn't common except in people with advanced disease, who may be fatigued, dizzy when they stand up, or have blood test abnormalities that are typical for this condition. **Cushing's syndrome** (excessive cortisol) can occur by combining PIs with certain steroid sprays (fluticasone, which is included in *Flonase* and *Advair*) or other forms of steroids (see Question 34). Taking steroids can make the adrenal glands "lazy," too, which can lead to adrenal insufficiency when the steroids are stopped.

Hypogonadism

A deficiency of testosterone, the male sex hormone.

Testosterone should only be used in men with low testosterone levels.

Testosterone

The male sex hormone, which can be low in some HIVpositive men.

Adrenal insufficiency

A deficiency in the amount of cortisol produced by the adrenal gland.

Adrenal gland

A gland in the abdomen that produces cortisol, a steroid hormone that is essential to many bodily functions, including the response to stress.

Cushing's syndrome

Excessive cortisol levels either because of overproduction by the adrenal glands or use of steroid medication.

Side Effects and Toxicity

52. Can ART affect my nervous system

The biggest risk to your nervous system is HIV itself. Untreated HIV infection can lead to a number of nasty neurologic problems, which are discussed further in Question 73. To prevent these problems, take ART. HIV drugs are pretty safe when it comes to the nervous system, but there are two things you should know about—toxic peripheral neuropathy and efavirenz side effects.

1. *Toxic peripheral neuropathy.* Stavudine (d4T, *Zerit*) and didanosine (ddI, *Videx*) can cause pain or numbness in the feet and legs (Question 45).
2. *Efavirenz side effects.* People who take efavirenz (*Sustiva, Atripla*) often experience *something* different with the first few doses—dizziness, vivid dreams (enjoyable or otherwise), and mental "fogginess" or difficulty concentrating, especially in the morning. These symptoms tend to get better with each dose and are often gone within a few days. If they last for more than 3 to 4 weeks they probably won't get better, and you may need to change medications. Here are some tips for getting used to efavirenz:
   A. Take it in the evening but at least 2 hours after dinner. Taking it with fatty food can increase drug levels and side effects.
   B. Don't take the first dose the night before you have something important to do. Wait until a weekend or a time when you have a few days off.
   C. If you're dreaming so much that you're not getting a good night's sleep, short-term use of a **benzodiazepine** (a tranquilizer in the *Valium* class) may help suppress the dreams.
   D. If you're too groggy in the morning, try taking it earlier in the evening.
   E. Once the side effects go away, you can take it however and whenever you want, as long as you take it each day. Rarely, efavirenz causes more severe psychiatric symptoms, such as depression or hallucinations. If you

Benzodiazepine

A class of drugs used to treat anxiety and insomnia.

find yourself depressed or hearing voices for the first time in your life after recently starting efavirenz, it's time to change drugs. Long-term effects can occur, too. If you're just "not yourself" (in terms of mood or ability to think or focus), talk to your provider about whether efavirenz could be the cause. Sometimes the only way to find out is to switch to a different drug and see what happens.

PART NINE

Opportunistic Infections and Other Complications

What are opportunistic infections?

How do I prevent or treat tuberculosis?

Can HIV cause cancer?

More . . .

53. What are opportunistic infections?

An "opportunist" is a person who takes advantage of opportunities, usually at the expense of others, for his own benefit. Similarly, an opportunistic infection (OI) is one in which a **pathogen** (a bacterium, virus, fungus, or parasite) takes advantage of a weakness in the body's defense mechanisms to cause disease. In the case of HIV infection, an OI is an infection caused by an organism that is normally kept in check by the **cellular immune system** (the part of the immune system that is most damaged by the HIV virus)*.

Some pathogens are exclusively opportunistic, meaning that they almost never cause problems in people with normal immune systems. Examples include many of the common HIV-related OIs, including *Pneumocystis*, *Cryptococcus*, *Mycobacterium avium complex* (**MAC**), and *Toxoplasma*. Other pathogens take advantage of immunosuppressed patients but can cause disease in anyone. Examples are **herpes simplex virus (HSV)**, human papilloma virus (HPV), and the bacterium that causes **tuberculosis**, each of which causes more frequent or severe disease in people with low CD4 counts. As a general rule, "exclusive opportunists" cause disease in people with lower CD4 counts than "optional opportunists."

In some cases, OIs can be prevented by avoiding exposure to the pathogen itself. For example, we lower the risk of spreading TB by isolating those who are actively infected; you can avoid toxoplasmosis by cooking meat properly; you can avoid syphilis by wearing condoms. However, many opportunistic pathogens are "ubiquitous"—they're found everywhere and can't be avoided. Examples include *Pneumocystis*, MAC, and *Cryptococcus*. Prevention of infections caused by these organisms requires either prophylaxis (medical treatment that prevents disease) or better yet, ART, which keeps the CD4 count above the danger zone.

*As opposed to the **humoral immune system**, which fights infections using antibodies.

An OI is an infection caused by an organism that is normally kept in check by the cellular immune system.

Pathogen

An infectious organism (bacterium, virus, fungus, or parasite) that causes disease.

Cellular immune system

The part of the immune system most directly affected by HIV infection. It controls a variety of bacterial, viral, fungal, and parasitic infections.

Pneumocystis

A fungus (*Pneumocystis jiroveci*) that is a common cause of pneumonia (PCP) in people with HIV infection.

Michael's comment:
After I was diagnosed, I assumed that anything and everything was a symptom of HIV. A cough? It's PCP. Tired after a sleepless night? HIV fatigue. I self-diagnosed thrush and ex-amined my lymph nodes daily. (Not that I knew where they were or what they were supposed to feel like.) If I stumbled, it was a sure sign of nerve trouble. Looking up into the daytime sky to follow the "floaters" was a daily test to self-diagnose CMV retinitis. I wasted many a beautiful summer afternoon that way. I can look back at those days now and smile, if not laugh.

Table 5 lists most of the complications of HIV infection and the CD4 counts at which they occur.

54. What is PCP?

PCP used to stand for *Pneumocystis carinii* pneumonia, one of the most common OIs in HIV-positive patients. *Pneumocystis* started out as a parasite, but people with too much time on their hands later decided it was a fungus and then changed the name to *Pneumocystis jiroveci*. However, they knew there would be a revolt if they changed the abbreviation to PJP, so they kept the PCP abbreviation, which now stands for ***Pneumocystis* p**neumonia.

You can't avoid being exposed to *Pneumocystis*. In fact, it may live harmlessly in our lungs already, causing problems only if we become immunosuppressed. You're unlikely to get PCP if your CD4 count is above 200.

The most common symptoms of PCP are gradually worsening shortness of breath, fever, and dry cough. Chest pain and yucky sputum are more typical of bacterial pneumonia, which tends to come on more suddenly.

PCP can be fatal if untreated—it was a common cause of death before we had effective treatment for HIV infection.

Cryptococcus

A fungus or yeast that is a common cause of meningitis in people with HIV infection.

Mycobacterium avium complex (MAC)

A bacterium related to tuberculosis that causes disease in people with advanced HIV disease, including fever, night sweats, weight loss, diarrhea, liver disease, abdominal pain, and anemia.

Herpes simplex virus (HSV)

A virus that causes painful blisters and ulcers on the lips, genitals, near the anus, or other parts of the skin.

PCP

Pneumocystis pneumonia, one of the most common OIs in an HIV-positive patient.

PCP can be fatal if untreated—it was a common cause of death before we had effective treatment for HIV infection.

Table 5 Complications of HIV Infection Based on CD4 Count		
CD4 count*	Infectious Complications	Noninfectious Complications
Above 500	Acute retroviral syndrome [11, 16]** Vaginal candidiasis [74]	Persistent generalized lymphadenopathy (PGL) [11] Guillain-Barré syndrome [16] Myopathy [16] Aseptic meningitis [16]
200-500	Bacterial pneumonia [66] Pulmonary tuberculosis [59] Shingles (herpes zoster) [70] Oral candidiasis (thrush) [63] Cryptosporidiosis, acute [65,91] Kaposi's sarcoma [61] Oral hairy leukoplakia (OHL) [63] Cervical and anal dysplasia or cancer [61,80]	Lymphoma [61] Anemia [69] Thrombocytopenia (low platelet count)
Less than 200	*Pneumocystis* pneumonia [54] Histoplasmosis or coccidioidomycosis [57] Tuberculosis involving organs other than the lungs [59] Progressive multifocal leukoencephalopathy (PML) [71, 72]	Weight loss and wasting [68] Peripheral neuropathy [72] HIV-associated dementia [72]
Less than 100	Toxoplasmosis [56] Cryptococcal meningitis [57] Cryptosporidiosis, chronic [65,91] Microsporidiosis [65] Candidal esophagitis [64]	
Less than 50	CMV disease [58] MAC infection [55]	Primary central nervous system lymphoma (PCNSL) [61]

*The conditions listed can occur at CD4 counts at or below the ranges shown on this table. Most become more frequent at lower CD4 counts. While uncommon, they can also occur at CD4 counts higher than the ranges listed.

**Numbers in brackets refer to Question numbers in this book.

Adapted with permission from Bartlett JG, Gallant JE. *2009-2010 Medical Management of HIV Infection*. Durham, NC: 2009 MMHIV, 2009.

Clues to the diagnosis include an abnormal chest x-ray and low oxygen levels in the blood. The diagnosis is made by an **induced sputum** exam, which involves inhaling a salt solution that makes you cough hard and deep, or **bronchoscopy**, where a flexible scope is used to sample fluid from your lungs. It's best to confirm the diagnosis since other conditions can look just like PCP, and side effects are common during the 3-week course of therapy.

The best treatment for PCP is trimethoprim-sulfa methoxazole (TMP-SMX, cotrimoxazole, *Bactrim, Septra*). There are alternatives for people who are allergic to sulfa drugs. People with severe PCP should also take prednisone, a steroid that keeps your breathing from getting worse before it gets better.

The best way to prevent PCP is to keep your CD4 count well above 200 with ART. Having an undetectable viral load helps too, regardless of your CD4 count. If your CD4 count is below 200, you should be on prophylaxis with low dose TMP-SMX or one of the alternatives. If your CD4 count rises above 200 for at least 3 months, you can talk to your provider about stopping prophylaxis. As with other OIs, PCP is much less common than it used to be thanks to effective ART.

55. What is MAC (MAI)?

MAC stands for *Mycobacterium avium* complex. It's also called **MAI**, for *Mycobacterium avium intracellulare*. It's a bacterium related to tuberculosis (TB), but unlike TB it rarely causes lung disease. Instead it infects the blood, causing fevers, chills, and night sweats. Given enough time, it can infect the bone marrow (causing anemia and low white blood cell counts), the liver (causing abnormal liver function tests), the wall of the intestines (causing wasting and diarrhea), and the lymph nodes (causing belly pain). In advanced HIV disease, MAC is disseminated, which means it's in the blood stream and spread throughout the body. To make a diagnosis of disseminated MAC, the organism should be grown in culture from

Induced sputum

A test used to diagnose PCP or tuberculosis in which patients inhale a saline mist that makes them cough deeply.

Bronchoscopy

A diagnostic procedure in which a flexible tube is inserted into the lungs through the mouth (under sedation) so that samples or biopsies can be taken.

The best way to prevent PCP is to keep your CD4 count well above 200 with ART.

a part of the body that's supposed to be sterile, such as blood, bone marrow, the liver, or other internal organs. MAC that's found in the sputum or the stool doesn't count as disseminated infection, as it may just be **colonizing** the intestines or lungs—present but not causing true disease.

Disseminated MAC requires treatment with either **clarithromycin** or **azithromycin** along with **ethambutol** and sometimes **rifabutin**. Treatment clears the blood and suppresses symptoms, but it's not a cure. MAC will return if the drugs are stopped. However, if your CD4 count increases on ART to above 100 for at least 6 months, you can talk to your provider about stopping MAC treatment.

MAC isn't a concern unless your CD4 count is below 50. Should you get to that point, you should take prophylaxis, either with weekly azithromycin, twice-daily clarithromycin, or daily rifabutin. Talk to your provider about stopping prophylaxis if your CD4 count rises above 100 for at least 3 months.

Like so many other OIs, you can't avoid exposure to MAC because it's everywhere. Prevention with ART or prophylaxis is the only way to prevent getting sick.

56. What is toxo?

"Toxo" is short for **toxoplasmosis**, a disease caused by the parasite *Toxoplasma gondii*. You get infected either by eating seriously undercooked meat (usually on purpose) or cat poop (usually by accident). After infection, the parasite lives in your body, walled off by the immune system, and causes no harm as long as your immune system remains healthy. However, if your CD4 count falls below 100, you can get sick. The most common and serious form of toxo is **encephalitis**, in which abscesses form in the brain.

A simple blood test, the **anti-*Toxoplasma* IgG antibody test**, will tell you whether you carry the parasite. A positive test means that at some time in your life you were infected. Perhaps as a child you shared a sandbox with Kitty or as an adult you developed a taste for carpaccio or steak tartar. If your test is positive, keep your CD4 count well above 100 with ART so your immune system can protect you. If it falls below 100, take prophylaxis, either with trimethoprim-sulfamethoxazole or with one of the alternatives to prevent encephalitis.

If you have a negative antibody test, avoid infection with the parasite. Don't eat raw or rare meat. Wear gloves in the garden, and wash your hands after digging in the dirt. Get someone else to change the litter box for you or use the appropriate precautions. There's no need to trade Kitty in for Fido if you're careful (see Question 94). Studies show no increased risk of toxo in cat owners.

Toxoplasmic encephalitis (also called CNS toxo) starts out with headache and/or neurologic symptoms such as seizures or weakness affecting one side of the body. It's treatable, but only with high doses of several unpleasant medications for at least 6 weeks, followed by lower doses for life (or until your CD4 count goes up with ART). Prevention is the way to go.

57. What about cryptococcal meningitis and other fungal infections?

Cryptococcal meningitis is an infection of the spinal fluid and lining of the brain with *Cryptococcus,* a yeast (fungus) that is found in the soil and inhaled into the lungs. Although people infected with *Cryptococcus* can develop pneumonia, skin lesions, or other symptoms, most people develop **meningitis** with gradually worsening headache and fever, sometimes with a stiff neck. Unlike bacterial meningitis, which makes you very sick very fast, crypto comes on more gradually. However, if left untreated it can lead to blindness, deafness, and even death. It's most likely to occur in people with CD4 counts below 100.

A simple blood test, the serum **cryptococcal antigen**, is almost always positive in people with cryptococcal meningitis. If the

Anti-*Toxoplasma* IgG antibody test

A blood test used to look for exposure to the *Toxoplasma* parasite.

Cryptococcal meningitis

Meningitis (infection of the spinal fluid and spinal cord lining) caused by *Cryptococcus.*

Meningitis

An infection or inflammation of the spinal fluid and the lining of the spinal cord.

Cryptococcal antigen

A lab test performed on either blood or spinal fluid used to diagnose cryptococcal meningitis.

Once you've been diagnosed with cryptococcal meningitis, you need to stay on fluconazole to prevent relapse.

test is positive you need a **spinal tap (lumbar puncture)** to confirm the diagnosis and to help determine the severity. Treatment usually involves at least 2 weeks of **amphotericin B** given by vein, often with **flucytosine (5-FC, *Ancobon*)**, followed by a long course of **fluconazole (*Diflucan*)**, given by mouth. In severe cases, frequent spinal taps may be needed to lower the spinal fluid pressure during the first few days of therapy. When people die of crypto, which isn't often, it's either because they waited too long to get treated or because they had high spinal fluid pressure that wasn't treated aggressively enough.

Once you've been diagnosed with cryptococcal meningitis, you need to stay on fluconazole to prevent **relapse** until your CD4 count has increased with ART (above 200 for at least 6 months). Since cryptococcal meningitis is easily treatable, unlikely to cause death if treated promptly, and less common than other OIs, we don't usually use prophylaxis to prevent it. There's no clear way to prevent initial infection with *Cryptococcus* since it's such a common organism.

While we're on the subject of serious fungal infections, it's worth mentioning a few more. **Candidiasis** is discussed in Questions 64, 65, and 75. **Histoplasmosis** is caused by *Histoplasma capsulatum*, a fungus that's common in the Ohio and Mississippi River Valleys. **Coccidioidomycosis ("cocci")** is caused by *Coccidioides immitis*, a fungus found in the valleys and deserts of the Southwestern United States and northern Mexico. Both can cause lung disease in people with normal immune systems, but they can cause more severe, widespread disease, including meningitis, in people with low CD4 counts. You can get infected by inhaling contaminated dust, and the fungus can live in your body and wait until your CD4 count is low to cause disease. If you're driving through Indianapolis or the San Joaquin Valley, hold your breath!

58. What is CMV?

Cytomegalovirus (CMV) means "big cell virus," because cells infected with CMV are big. CMV is a type of **herpesvirus**, and like all herpesviruses, you don't get rid of it once you've got it. Since it's common and easily transmitted sexually, most people with HIV infection have already been exposed to it and have been infected.

CMV is rarely a problem for people with normal immune systems, including HIV-positive people with even moderate CD4 counts. You only have to worry about CMV when your CD4 count drops below 50. The most common complication of CMV is **retinitis**, an infection of the retina (the back of the eye), which can lead to blindness if not treated. Report visual changes to your doctor *immediately* if you have a low CD4 count. If your CD4 count is below 100, you should be seeing an ophthalmologist for screening at least once or twice a year.

CMV can also cause gastrointestinal problems, including painful ulcers in the esophagus (**esophagitis**) (Question 64), or infection of the stomach (**gastritis**), small intestines (**enteritis**) or colon (**colitis**) causing diarrhea and abdominal pain. CMV can also affect the nervous system, causing infection of the brain (encephalitis), the spinal cord (**myelitis**), or the spinal nerves (**radiculitis**, **radiculopathy**).

A positive **anti-CMV IgG** antibody test means you've got the virus. There's not much to do about it other than to keep your CD4 count above 50. If the test is negative, then avoid CMV infection. Practice safe sex, and if you should ever need a transfusion, it should be with CMV-negative blood.

59. How do I prevent or treat tuberculosis?

Anyone can get tuberculosis (TB), but the risk is much higher for HIV-positive people, and it increases as the CD4 count falls. People with low CD4 counts can get more severe forms

The most common complication of CMV is retinitis, an infection of the retina (the back of the eye), which can lead to blindness if not treated.

Histoplasmosis

A disease caused by *Histoplasma capsulatum*, a fungus found mostly in the Ohio and Mississippi River valleys, which causes lung infection in people with normal immune systems, and infection of the lungs and other organs in people with low CD4 counts.

Coccidioidomycosis ("cocci")

A disease cause by *Coccidioides immitis*, a fungus found mostly in the deserts and valleys of the southwestern United States and northern Mexico.

Cytomegalovirus (CMV)

A virus that can infect the eyes, the gastrointestinal tract, the liver, and the nervous system in people with advanced HIV.

of TB, which can spread throughout the body, involving organs other than the lungs. You become infected with *Mycobacterium tuberculosis* (the TB bacterium) through close contact with someone who has active TB and is coughing. Infection doesn't always lead to illness. Your body may be able to control the organism on its own, especially if you have a high CD4 count. But if the CD4 count falls, your immune system may no longer be able to protect you, and you may get sick.

Everyone with HIV should be tested for TB infection either with a tuberculin skin test (TST, also known as a PPD) or an interferon-gamma release assay (IGRA) blood test. A positive test doesn't mean you have TB, but it usually means you've been exposed to the organism and are at risk for getting sick. If you've *ever* had a positive test, have been in close contact with someone with active TB, or if there's evidence of old TB on your chest x-ray, you should take a 9-month course of **isoniazid (INH)** to kill the bacteria and prevent TB. Shorter courses of therapy using two drugs may be recommended soon. These tests may not be accurate if you're immunosuppressed, so they should be repeated after your CD4 count has increased due to ART.

Symptoms of active TB include prolonged fever, night sweats, weight loss, and cough with yucky or bloody sputum; other symptoms depend on the parts of the body involved. The diagnosis is usually made with sputum tests, though bronchoscopy or biopsies of the affected organs may sometimes be necessary. TB is curable with a 6-month course of therapy involving a combination of drugs. Because it's so contagious, treatment is managed by the health department, using **directly observed therapy (DOT)**.

60. When do I need OI prophylaxis?

Prophylaxis is a fancy term for prevention. When we talk about prophylaxis, we're generally referring to the use of a drug to prevent an opportunistic infection (OI). If your viral

---

Anyone can get tuberculosis (TB), but the risk is much higher for HIV-positive people.

Herpesvirus
A family of viruses that can cause acute infection but that also remain latent in the body and recur.

Retinitis
An infection of the retina (the interior surface of the back of the eye) which can lead to blindness if not treated. Most often caused by CMV.

Esophagitis
Infection or inflammation of the esophagus.

Gastritis
Infection or inflammation of the stomach.

Enteritis
Infection or inflammation of the small intestines.

Colitis
Infection or inflammation of the colon (large intestine).

Myelitis
Infection or inflammation of the spinal cord.

load is undetectable and your CD4 count is high, there's not much you need to worry about. If your CD4 count is low here's what you can do to prevent some OIs:

- *PCP.* Start prophylaxis with trimethoprim/sulfamethoxazole (TMP-SMX, *Bactrim*, *Septra*) when your CD4 count is less than 200. If you can't take TMP/SMX use **dapsone**, and if you can't take that use **aerosolized pentamidine** or **atovaquone (*Mepron*)** (Question 54).
- *Toxoplasmosis.* Start prophylaxis if you have a positive anti-*Toxoplasma* IgG antibody *and* your CD4 count is less than 100. If you're already taking TMP/SMX, you're covered (but make sure you're taking a double strength tablet daily). If you can't take TMP/SMX, use a combination of dapsone, **pyrimethamine (*Daraprim*)**, and **leucovorin (folinic acid)**. If your antibody is negative, avoid exposure (Questions 56 and 94).
- *Mycobacterium avium complex (MAC).* Start prophylaxis if your CD4 count is less than 50. Use azithromycin 1,200 mg per week or clarithromycin 500 mg twice a day (Question 55).
- *Cytomegalovirus (CMV).* Prophylaxis isn't recommended. Most people with HIV infection have already been exposed and are at risk for getting sick only if their CD4 count falls below 50 (Question 58).
- *Fungal infections (*Candida and *cryptococcal meningitis).* Unless you've already had one of these infections, prophylaxis isn't recommended (Question 57).
- *Herpes and shingles.* If you've never had these problems, prevention is not recommended. If you have frequent bouts of herpes (several per year), consider chronic suppression with **acyclovir (*Zovirax*)**, **valacyclovir (*Valtrex*)**, or **famciclovir (*Famvir*)**. Shingles doesn't usually strike more than once, but when it does, prophylaxis is sometimes necessary (Question 89).

Opportunistic Infections and Other Complications

Radiculitis (radiculopathy)

Infection or inflammation of the nerves that emerge from the spinal cord.

Anti-CMV IgG

A blood test used to look for infection with CMV.

Isoniazid (INH)

A drug used to treat or prevent tuberculosis.

Directly observed therapy (DOT)

A program in which treat-ment is given to a patient directly by a healthcare professional, at home or in a clinic, in order to ensure that it's taken.

Dapsone

A drug used to treat or prevent PCP and to prevent toxoplasmosis.

Aerosolized pentamidine

A drug used to prevent PCP.

Atovaquone (*Mepron*)

A drug used to treat or prevent PCP.

Pyrimethamine (*Daraprim*)

A drug used to treat or prevent PCP or toxoplasmosis.

Leucovorin (folinic acid)

A drug used to prevent bone marrow toxicity due to pyrimethamine.

Acyclovir (Zovirax)

A drug used to treat herpes simplex and varicella zoster virus.

Valacyclovir (Valtrex)

A drug used to treat herpes simplex and varicella zoster virus.

Famciclovir (Famvir)

A drug used to treat herpes simplex and varicella zoster virus.

Kaposi's sarcoma (KS).

A tumor caused by a virus that is more common in people with HIV infection, especially gay men.

Human herpesvirus-8 (HHV-8)

The virus that causes Kaposi's sarcoma, Castleman's syndrome, and some rare lymphomas.

Kaposi's sarcoma-associated herpesvirus (KSHV)

A tumor caused by a virus that is more common in people with HIV infection, especially gay men.

61. Can HIV cause cancer?

People with HIV infection are at increased risk for certain cancers, though they're still far less common than OIs. The cancers most strongly associated with HIV infection are discussed below.

- **Kaposi's sarcoma (KS)** was a huge problem during the early years of the epidemic; fortunately, we see a lot less of it now. It's caused by a virus, human **herpesvirus-8 (HHV-8)**, also known as **Kaposi's sarcoma-associated herpesvirus (KSHV)**. For reasons that aren't completely understood, KS occurs mostly in gay and bisexual men. It typically causes raised, purple-colored skin lesions, but it can also affect the mouth, lungs, GI tract, and other organs. Mild cases can be treated with topical therapies applied to the skin lesions themselves, but more severe cases need to be treated with cancer chemotherapy. Although it often gets better with HIV therapy, KS can sometimes occur even with high CD4 counts.

- **Lymphoma** doesn't happen often, but it's a serious problem when it occurs. The most common type is **non-Hodgkin's lymphoma (NHL)**, but people with HIV infection also have an increased risk of **Hodgkin's disease** and **Burkitt's lymphoma**. Lymphoma can pop up just about anywhere in the body and is diagnosed by taking a piece of abnormal tissue (**biopsy**). It responds very well to chemotherapy, but the outcome depends on the CD4 count. Being on effective ART helps a lot.

- **Primary central nervous system lymphoma (PCNSL)**, a lymphoma of the brain, is the cancer you'd *least* want to have. Fortunately, it almost never happens in people with CD4 counts above 50. It's treated with radiation, but in the bad old days, the prognosis was miserable. Things are a little better now—still, this is something to be avoided by taking ART.

- **Cervical cancer and anal cancer** are caused by human papillomavirus (HPV), a sexually transmitted virus that causes dysplasia (abnormal cells), which can eventually turn into cancer if not treated. Women should get regular Pap smears to diagnose dysplasia and prevent cancer. **Anal Pap smears** are now being done, too, especially for women and gay and bisexual men, though straight men can get anal HPV infection, as well. This isn't a standard test yet, but it may become one. For more on HPV-related cancers, see Question 81.

I've discussed the most common HIV-related cancers, but it's possible that HIV-positive people may be at higher risk for some of the more "garden variety" cancers as well. Being on ART probably helps; starting it early may help even more. Make sure you're up-to-date on standard age-based cancer screening tests (colonoscopy, mammogram, PSA, etc.).

62. What is immune reconstitution?

Immune reconstitution refers to the repair of the immune system with ART. It's usually a good thing, except when it leads to the **immune reconstitution inflammatory syndrome (IRIS)**, in which the body's newly restored ability to fight infections creates problems.

Let's use MAC as an example (Question 55). You don't get MAC unless your immune system is severely damaged, usually with a CD4 count below 50. At that point, your immune system is completely incapable of fighting off the bacteria that are running rampant in the body. However, if you start ART when you have MAC, your immune system may recover enough to start doing its job. It may try to form walls around the bacteria, leading to abscesses or enlarged, inflamed lymph nodes. The immune response may cause fever, night sweats, and weight loss.

Cervical cancer and anal cancer are caused by human papillomavirus (HPV), a sexually transmitted virus that causes dysplasia (abnormal cells)

Lymphoma

A cancer of the lymphatic tissue that is more common in people with HIV infection.

Non-Hodgkin's lymphoma (NHL)

The most common type of lymphoma in people with HIV infection.

Hodgkin's disease

A type of lymphoma that is more common in people with HIV but is less common than non-Hodgkin's lymphoma (NHL).

Burkitt's lymphoma

A type of lymphoma that is seen more frequently in people with HIV infection but is less common than non-Hodgkin's lymphoma (NHL).

Biopsy

A procedure in which a piece of tissue is removed, either with a needle through the skin, through a scope placed in the lungs or gastrointestinal tract, or by a surgical procedure.

Primary central nervous system lymphoma (PCNSL)

A lymphoma involving the brain, seen only in people with advanced HIV disease.

Cervical cancer

A cancer of the cervix (the mouth of the uterus) caused by human papillomavirus (HPV).

Anal cancer

A cancer of the anus caused by human papillomavirus (HPV).

Anal Pap smears

A diagnostic test to screen for anal dysplasia.

IRIS can occur with a variety of organisms. The most common are MAC and TB, but it can also happen with CMV, PCP, *Cryptococcus*, and others. People sometimes have outbreaks of shingles or herpes after they start ART. Even Kaposi's sarcoma and **progressive multifocal leukoencphalopathy (PML)**, which usually get better with ART, can sometimes get worse.

As unpleasant as IRIS can be, it's temporary and a sign that your immune system is recovering. In almost all cases, you should continue ART. It's important to find out what the underlying OI is, usually with a biopsy, and then treat it. Steroids (prednisone) are sometimes used to help get people through IRIS by blunting the immune response to the organism while still allowing ART to suppress HIV. The prednisone dose can be gradually lowered until the symptoms are gone.

63. Will HIV or ART make me age faster?

There's been a lot of talk recently about "accelerated aging" with HIV infection. The term is scary and a little misleading. It doesn't mean that the overall aging process is being sped up and that you're on a faster pace to the grave. Instead, it refers to the fact that some of the complications of aging are being seen at younger ages in some HIV-positive people. Examples include heart disease, decreased bone density, risk of cancer, and changes in brain function, including dementia.

There are many unanswered questions about HIV and aging, which is now the subject of a great deal of speculation as well as scientific research:

1. *Is premature aging caused by HIV, ART or both?* HIV itself itself is mostly to blame. There is evidence that people who start ART with low CD4 counts are at greater risk for heart disease, bone fractures, and cognitive impairment (brain disease). People who spend a lot of time

with high viral loads are at greater risk of lymphoma and other complications. It's clear that early effective ART goes a long way toward preventing the long-term complications of HIV, but ART isn't completely off the hook, since treatment with some drugs may increase the risk of kidney disease, loss of bone density, and atherosclerosis. We do know that ART does a lot more good than harm.

2. *How does HIV accelerate aging?* I've talked before about the inflammation and immune activation that occur with HIV infection (Question 9). These are the most likely reasons for the increased risk of aging complications. ART dramatically reduces these processes, which explains many of its long-term benefits.

3. *Can HIV cause premature aging despite effective ART?* ART clearly helps to slow this process, but we don't know whether taking ART early in the course of HIV infection, starting at a high CD4 count, will completely eliminate the long-term risks. People on ART have much lower levels of inflammation and immune activation than people who aren't being treated, but their levels are still higher than those of HIV-negative people. We'll need more time to find out whether someone with optimally treated HIV infection can expect the same lifespan and quality of life as someone without HIV infection.

We have much to learn about the effects of HIV infection and ART on aging. I hope to have a lot more to tell you in the next edition of this book. In the meantime, the best way to stay healthy into your old age is to keep your viral load suppressed on ART (while not forgetting all of the other things we're all told to do to become healthy, vigorous senior citizens).

Immune reconstitution inflammatory syndrome (IRIS)

A condition that sometimes occurs in people with low CD4 counts who start ART in which the improved immune system reacts to organisms (such as MAC, the TB bacterium, or fungi), causing illness, including fevers, weight loss, swollen lymph nodes, or abscesses.

Progressive multifocal leuko-encphalopathy (PML)

An infection of the brain caused by JC virus, which results in progressive neurologic deterioration.

Opportunistic Infections and Other Complications

PART TEN

Symptoms

What can I do about nausea and diarrhea?

What if I get a cold or the flu?

Why am I so tired?

More . . .

Oropharyngeal candidiasis

Candida (yeast) infection involving the mouth and throat, including thrush, angular cheilitis, and erythematous candidiasis.

Candida

A fungus (yeast) that can cause thrush, esophagitis, and vaginitis in people with HIV infection.

Oral hairy leukoplakia (OHL)

Painless white plaques, or "stripes," on the sides of the tongue caused by Epstein-Barr virus.

Epstein-Barr virus (EBV)

A herpesvirus that causes infectious mononucleosis ("mono"), oral hairy leukoplakia, and some lymphomas.

Thrush and OHL are fairly benign conditions, but they both indicate that something's seriously wrong with your immune system and that you should be on ART.

---

64. What's wrong with my mouth?

The most common cause of mouth and throat problems is **oropharyngeal candidiasis** ("thrush"), a buildup of *Candida* (a common yeast or fungus). Thrush is easy to diagnose with a mirror and a flashlight. You'll see whitish-yellow curd-like patches, especially on the roof and sides of the mouth, the back of the throat, and the gums. These patches can be easily scraped off. Don't confuse a white coating on the tongue with thrush. The tongue is usually the last part of the mouth to be infected, and a white coating on the tongue, with no other evidence of thrush, is usually just. . .a white coating on the tongue.

Thrush can also be confused with **oral hairy leukoplakia (OHL),** a condition caused by **Epstein-Barr virus (EBV)** that looks like a white racing stripe down both sides of the tongue. Unlike thrush, it can't be scraped off. *Candida* can cause other mouth problems besides thrush—**erythematous candidiasis** (redness on the roof of the mouth that is sometimes painful) and **angular cheilitis** (cracks at the corners of the lips).

Painful ulcers in the mouth can be caused by viruses, but they're more often **aphthous ulcers,** which essentially means that we have no idea what causes them. The diagnosis of most of these conditions is usually based on appearance alone; special tests aren't necessary.

Thrush and OHL are fairly benign conditions, but they both indicate that something's seriously wrong with your immune system and that you should be on ART. Thrush is treated with antifungal medication. Fluconazole, an oral antifungal drug, is very effective, but repeated use can lead to infection with drug-resistant fungus, which is why we sometimes use medications that treat only the surfaces, such as **clotrimazole troches** (lozenges) or **nystatin** mouth rinses. Because it's harmless, we don't usually treat OHL except with ART.

Before we leave the mouth, don't forget your teeth and gums. People with low CD4 counts are at risk for serious mouth infections. Brushing, flossing, and seeing a dentist and oral hygienist on a regular basis are important to keep your teeth and gums in good shape.

65. Why does it hurt to swallow?

There are two medical terms for swallowing symptoms—**dysphagia** (difficulty swallowing) and **odynophagia** (painful swallowing), but the distinction is less important than the location. Is the problem confined to the back of the throat (**pharynx**) or does it extend into the chest (**esophagus**)? For mouth and throat symptoms, see Question 64.

When the problem is in the chest, it can be a sign of esophagitis, an inflammation of the esophagus, the tube that connects your throat with your stomach. The most common cause is *Candida*, the same yeast (fungus) that causes thrush and **vaginitis**. People with *Candida* esophagitis usually have a CD4 count below 100. Since *Candida* is the most common cause of esophagitis, the usual approach is to treat with fluconazole and see what happens. If *Candida* is the cause, you'll be swallowing easier within a day or two. If not, you'll need an **endoscopy**, an outpatient procedure in which a flexible tube with a camera is passed from the mouth into the esophagus so that pictures and biopsies can be taken.

Other causes of esophagitis are herpes simplex virus (HSV), cytomegalovirus (CMV), and aphthous ulcers, each of which causes painful ulcers in the wall of the esophagus. The treatment of these conditions depends on the cause. Drug-resistant *Candida* can also cause esophagitis and must be treated with other antifungal drugs.

Of course, HIV-positive people can also develop the same esophageal problems that HIV-negative people get, including esophageal reflux, spasm, or strictures. Pills can get stuck on

Symptoms

Erythematous candidiasis

An infection of the mouth caused by *Candida* in which the roof of the mouth (palate) becomes red and sometimes painful.

Aphthous ulcers

Painful ulcers in the mouth (aphthous stomatitis) or esophagus (aphthous esophagitis) that can occur in people with HIV.

Clotrimazole troches

Antifungal lozenges used to treat thrush.

Nystatin

An antifungal mouth rinse used to treat thrush.

Dysphagia

Difficulty swallowing.

Candida is the most common cause of esophagitis.

Odynophagia

Painful swallowing.

Pharynx

Throat.

Esophagus

The tube that connects the mouth and throat to the stomach.

Vaginitis

Infection or inflammation of the vagina.

Endoscopy

A medical procedure in which a flexible tube is inserted into the esophagus and stomach through the mouth, while the patient is sedated, in order to take samples or biopsies or to treat a variety of conditions.

Cryptosporidiosis

Diarrhea caused by *Cryptosporidium*, a parasite that can be found in contaminated water or transmitted from person to person.

Microsporidia

A variety of opportunistic parasites that cause chronic diarrhea in people with low CD4 counts.

Salmonella

A group of bacteria that can cause severe diarrhea, fever, and bloodstream infections.

Colonoscopy

A medical procedure in which a flexible scope is inserted into the rectum and colon through the anus, while the patient is sedated, in order to look for abnormalities and take biopsies.

the way down and irritate the esophagus, so always take your meds with plenty of water.

66. What can I do about nausea and diarrhea?

In HIV-positive people, nausea is most often caused by medications. Zidovudine (AZT, *Retrovir, Combivir, Trizivir*) and some of the protease inhibitors are the most common offenders. If your nausea began as soon as you started a new drug, then there's no mystery about the cause. In some cases, the nausea may improve with time or by taking the pills with food. Your doctor can also prescribe medications for nausea, but if the problem persists, you may have to change drugs. If you've developed nausea but haven't recently changed or added medications, then it's important to look further for a cause.

Diarrhea can be caused by medications, too, especially some of the older PIs. The best way to treat drug-related diarrhea is with daily fiber supplements, such as psyllium. Don't be put off by the word "laxative" on the bottle. Fiber supplements add bulk to the stool, which is a good thing whether you've got diarrhea or constipation. If they don't work, ask your doctor about prescribed or over-the-counter anti-diarrhea medications, or about making a change in your regimen.

There are many infectious causes of diarrhea, including common viruses, bacteria, and parasites. Some of these organisms, such as *Cryptosporidium* (which causes **cryptosporidiosis**), **microsporidia**, *Isospora* (which causes **isoporiasis**), and *Salmonella* are opportunistic—they occur or are more severe because of immunosuppression. Advanced HIV infection itself can also cause diarrhea. If you have prolonged diarrhea that's not caused by medications, you'll need to be evaluated, first with stool studies, and if those are negative, with a scope (flexible tube with a camera), either from above (endoscopy), from below (**colonoscopy**), or both.

Diarrhea caused by viruses or food poisoning usually gets better on its own after a few days, but get medical attention if you have persistent diarrhea, or if you have fever, belly pain, blood in your stool, or dizziness. When you have diarrhea, eat a bland diet with no milk products, and hydrate, hydrate, hydrate!

> *Michael's comment:*
> *Fiber supplements work. They work for diarrhea caused by PIs, and they work for constipation caused by calcium supplements. Some types are more palatable and work better than others. The one I am using these days is right tasty. I take it with both my morning and evening meds. Neither the capsules nor the chewables work as well for me as the powder that I add to a glass of water. I have found a few brands that I like, and I switch between flavors before I get too sick of any one. When I skip a serving, I can tell the difference, and the change isn't for the better.*

67. What do I do about cough or shortness of breath?

The possible causes of cough or shortness of breath depend on your CD4 count. If it's well above 200, then the list is about the same as it would be in an HIV-negative person. Cough can be due to the common cold, bronchitis, pneumonia, asthma, smoking, the use of certain medications, or esophageal reflux (stomach acid going up into the esophagus rather than staying in the stomach). Shortness of breath can be due to asthma, pneumonia, anemia, or acidosis (a buildup of acid in your blood). The kind of cough you get with a common cold or bronchitis doesn't usually require medical attention (Question 68). If you recently had a cold and now have one of those nagging, hacking coughs that gets worse when you laugh, exercise, or go out in the cold, you may have **bronchospasm (or reactive airways)**, which can be treated with an inhaled bronchodilator.

Bronchospasm (or reactive airways)

The tendency of the bronchi (airways in the lung) to constrict (narrow), causing shortness of breath or cough.

Symptoms

The same is true if your CD4 count is low, except that now there's a longer list of possible causes. If your count is below 200, you may have PCP (Question 54). With a count less than 100, there's a risk for pneumonia caused by *Cryptococcus*, *Toxoplasma*, or *Histoplasma*, which are less common than PCP. HIV-positive people are at much higher risk for TB at any CD4 count, and the risk gets higher as the CD4 gets lower (Question 59).

You should never ignore shortness of breath or any change in your ability to exert yourself.

You should get medical attention if you have a severe cough or one that doesn't get better with time, or if you have a high fever, chest pain when you take a deep breath, or are coughing up blood. You should never ignore shortness of breath or any change in your ability to exert yourself. If you're winded after climbing one flight of stairs but could climb three flights a month ago, you need to get checked out.

68. What do I o if I get a cold or the flu?

HIV-positive people get colds and flu just like everyone else. The symptoms and duration of the illness are the same, and they're at no greater risk from complications. That's because viruses that cause the cold and flu are controlled by the **humoral** (antibody-mediated) **immune system**, not the cellular immune system that uses CD4 cells and is damaged by HIV.

Humoral immune system

The part of the immune system that uses antibodies to fight infection.

For that reason, you don't need to do anything special if you get a cold—just rest and drink plenty of fluids. The usual over-the-counter cold remedies are safe and don't interact with HIV drugs. *You don't need antibiotics just because you're positive.* Your illness is caused by a virus; antibiotics kill only bacteria. They're often prescribed as placebos to keep people happy, but that's creating a big drug resistance problem. If we want to have antibiotics around to treat serious bacterial infections, we need to stop using them to treat viral infections that get better on their own.

It *is* appropriate to use antibiotics in certain situations:

1. **Strep throat**. The diagnosis requires a culture or rapid strep screen—there's no other way to tell the difference between strep throat and the more common type of sore throat caused by cold viruses. Antibiotics don't make strep throat get better faster; they just decrease the risk of rare complications, such as rheumatic fever.
2. **Sinusitis.** See Question 72 for symptoms. In addition to antibiotics, don't forget the decongestants. The use of decongestants during a cold may keep your sinuses draining and prevent tsinusitis from happening.
3. **Pneumonia**. See Question 67 for symptoms.

Studies have shown that **bronchitis** doesn't get better any faster with antibiotics. Cough medicine and sometimes an inhaled bronchodilator may help you feel better, but as with the common cold, you just have to ride it out.

For true influenza during flu season, the use of anti-influenza drugs can shorten the course of the illness, but only if used within the first few days.

69. Why am I losing weight?

During the dark days before ART, weight loss was almost universal as AIDS progressed, and many patients wasted away to nothing before they died. Weight loss is much less common now that we have effective therapy for HIV infection. Here are some common, treatable causes of weight loss:

1. *Untreated HIV infection.* If you're losing weight because of HIV infection, you need to be on ART. Weight loss is more likely to occur if you have a high viral load.
2. *Hypogonadism.* Men with low testosterone levels can lose weight (Question 51). Check your thyroid function while you're at it with a TSH (thyroid stimulating hormone level).

Strep throat

The common term for streptococcal pharyngitis, a bacterial infection of the throat caused by group A beta-hemolytic *Streptococcus.*

Sinusitis

An infection of the sinuses; air spaces in the head connected to the nasal passages.

Pneumonia

An infection of the air spaces of the lungs, which can be caused by a variety of infectious organisms.

Bronchitis

An infection of the bronchi (airways), usually caused by a viral infection often after a common cold.

Symptoms

3. *Depression.* This is a common cause of weight loss, since depressed people often lose their appetites (Questions 82 and 83).
4. *Lipoatrophy.* This doesn't usually cause loss of total body weight, but it can make you look like you've lost weight (Question 46).
5. *Gastrointestinal disorders.* Problems in the esophagus could make it harder to swallow; nausea and vomiting could make you less likely to eat or to absorb your food; you could also have a problem with absorption of nutrients in the small intestine.

In the past, we often used anabolic steroids to help people gain muscle mass as they wasted away from AIDS. It wasn't a solution to the problem, but it helped control the symptoms. I don't see much wasting anymore, but I do see men who want to use their HIV status as an excuse to get big muscles without having to spend as much time at the gym. That's probably not a good idea. After all, if I were convinced that anabolic steroids were perfectly safe, *I'd* be ripped!

70. Why am I so tired?

Fatigue is common among HIV-positive people. If you're experiencing an unusual amount of fatigue, consider the following possible causes:

Anemia is easy to diagnose with a simple blood count.

Hypothyroidism

A deficiency in thyroid hormone.

- *Depression.* This may be the most common reason for fatigue. People with depression have no energy, but they also have a number of other symptoms, discussed in Question 82.
- *Anemia.* In addition to fatigue, people with anemia may be pale, dizzy, and short of breath. Causes include medications, especially zidovudine (AZT, *Retrovir, Combivir, Trizivir*), dietary deficiencies, HIV-related complications, and HIV itself. Anemia is easy to diagnose with a simple blood count.
- *Hormone deficiencies.* These include low testosterone levels (hypogonadism), thyroid hormone deficiency (**hypothyroidism**), and adrenal insufficiency (Question 51).

- *Medications.* Zidovudine is known to cause fatigue even when it's not causing anemia. Efavirenz (*Sustiva, Atripla*) can do it, too, especially in the first few weeks if it's disturbing your sleep with lots of wild dreams (Question 52).
- *Lactic acidosis.* This is an uncommon but serious side effect of stavudine (d4T, *Zerit*), zidovudine, and possibly didanosine (ddI, *Videx*). Lactic acidosis causes other symptoms as well, which are discussed in Question 45.
- *HIV infection.* Fatigue is common in people with high viral loads and/or low CD4 counts, or when there's significant wasting.

Since virtually all of the causes of fatigue are treatable, it's important to make the diagnosis. Fatigue is not something you should have to live with.

71. Can HIV affect my skin?

Skin problems can be caused by HIV itself, by complications of HIV, and by medications. It's hard to talk about skin problems in a book without color pictures, and I don't have room to talk about treatment. If you're having skin problems, see your provider or a dermatologist. Here's an incomplete list of things that can go wrong with the skin:

- **Abscesses** ("boils") have become common due to the epidemic of community acquired **methicillin-resistant Staph aureus (MRSA)**. They usually have to be opened up and drained. It's important to culture the pus first so that the right antibiotic can be chosen.
- Drug reactions often begin with a red, itchy rash. They can be caused by the NNRTIs, some PIs, especially fosamprenavir (*Lexiva*) and darunavir (*Prezista*), trimethoprim-sulfamethoxazole, and many other medications.
- **Folliculitis** causes raised, itchy, red bumps in areas where there's hair. It can be caused by bacteria, *Demodex* mites, or can be "eosinophilic," a term used to describe the type of cells that are seen on a biopsy.

Symptoms

Fatigue is not something you should have to live with.

Abscesses

Collections of pus (infectious organisms and white blood cells) in the skin ("boil") or other parts of the body.

Methicillin-resistant *Staphylococcus aureus* (MRSA)

A drug-resistant bacterium that traditionally caused serious illness in seriously ill hospitalized patients but that has recently become a common cause of skin disease, including abscesses (community-acquired MRSA).

Folliculitis

Infection of the hair follicles and skin around them.

Molluscum contagiosum

Flesh-colored bumps or protuberances on the skin that are caused by a poxvirus and can be sexually transmitted.

Bartonella

A bacterium that can cause skin disease (bacillary angiomatosis) or liver disease (peliosis hepatis) in people with HIV.

Bacillary angiomatosis

A bacterial skin disease caused by Bartonella, which causes raised purple lesions on the skin sometimes confused with Kaposi's sarcoma.

Prurigo nodularis

A condition characterized by itchy bumps on the skin, seen more commonly in people with HIV.

Psoriasis

A skin condition that results in dry, scaly, itchy plaques on the skin that can get worse with immunosuppression due to HIV infection.

Scabies

An itchy skin condition caused by a mite that burrows under the skin and can be spread to others by close contact.

- Herpes simplex can affect the lips, the genitals, the area around the anus, or other parts of the skin. It causes small, painful blisters that open up and become shallow ulcers on a red base.
- Kaposi's sarcoma causes raised purple lesions on the skin or in the mouth (Question 61).
- **Molluscum contagiosum** lesions are raised, skin-colored, fleshy bumps with small indentations in the middle. They can occur anywhere but are especially common on the genitals, face, and neck.
- Opportunistic infections can cause skin problems, including cryptococcosis, histoplasmosis, and **Bartonella** (**bacillary angiomatosis**). A skin biopsy is usually the best way to make the diagnosis.
- **Prurigo nodularis** means "itchy bumps" in Latin. This may be a reaction to too much scratching over a long period of time.
- **Psoriasis** can get worse, or appear for the first time, in people with low CD4 counts. It causes itchy raised patches, especially on the elbows, knees, and buttocks.
- **Scabies** is caused by a common skin mite. It causes intense itching, especially at night. A common location is on the backs of the hands and between the fingers. It can be quite extensive and severe in people with low CD4 counts.
- **Seborrheic dermatitis** causes a flaky, red rash on the face, especially in the folds on the cheeks and around the eyebrows.
- Secondary syphilis can cause a variety of rashes, including red bumps, sometimes involving the palms and soles (Question 88).
- Shingles is reactivation of varicella zoster virus (VZV), the chicken-pox virus, in the skin over a single nerve. It causes painful blisters in a confined, band-like area on one side of the body.

72. Why do I have a headache?

If your CD4 count is over 100 and you've got a headache, it's probably due to one of the usual causes—tension headache, migraine, or sinus headache. A **tension headache** feels like a band-like tightness or constriction, tends to come on later in the day, and is present on both sides of the head. A **migraine** can occur at any time of the day, is often present on one side of the head, may be throbbing, and may occur with visual changes or nausea. People with a **sinus headache** have sinus congestion, a feeling of fullness or pressure below the eyes or in the forehead, and lots of thick, yucky snot.

If your CD4 count is below 100 and you have a headache, especially a chronic headache that just gets gradually worse, possibly with fever or stiff neck, you should be checked for cryptococcal meningitis (Question 57). A simple blood test, the serum cryptococcal antigen, will tell you if cryptococcal meningitis is likely. If the test is positive, you need a spinal tap to confirm the diagnosis and to find out the severity. Other types of meningitis (bacterial, *Listeria*) are far less common but come on more suddenly. They can also start out with a headache and fever.

If you also have neurologic changes (seizures, weakness or numbness on one side of the body, coordination problems, or mental changes), you could have a mass in the brain, usually caused by either toxoplasmosis (Question 56) or a brain lymphoma (Question 61). The first step here is an MRI scan of the brain with contrast injected through the vein. Progressive multifocal leukoencephalopathy (PML), which is caused by **JC virus**, can also cause neurologic symptoms, but it's less likely to cause a headache.

If your CD4 count is below 100 and you have a headache, especially a chronic headache that just gets gradually worse, possibly with fever or stiff neck, you should be checked for cryptococcal meningitis.

Symptoms

Seborrheic dermatitis

A common skin condition causing flakiness on the face, especially around the eyebrows and in the folds on the cheeks.

Tension headache

A headache caused by muscle tension.

Migraine headache

A severe headache, often on one side of the head, sometimes accompanied by visual changes or nausea.

Sinus headache

A headache caused by congestion of the sinuses.

Listeria

A foodborne bacterium that can cause meningitis and other infections.

JC virus

The cause of progressive multifocal leukoencephalopathy (PML).

The most common cause of memory loss is depression, which can sometimes look very much like dementia.

Neuro-psychological testing

A series of tests, usually performed by a psychologist or neurologist, to assess memory and thinking skills.

73. Can HIV affect my nervous system?

Untreated HIV infection is bad for your nervous system. The virus gets into the brain and spinal fluid and can lead to a lot of unpleasant complications. The way to prevent these problems is to take ART. I'll discuss the approach to some neurologic symptoms here.

- *Headache.* See Question 72.
- *Memory loss or personality changes.* The most common cause of memory loss is depression, which can sometimes look very much like dementia. It's possible to tell the difference with special memory and thinking tests (**neuropsychological testing**), but if there's any question, a few weeks of treatment with an antidepressant can help sort it out (Questions 81 and 82). If you're experiencing memory loss but aren't depressed, then it's important to find out whether you have HIV dementia or other HIV-related brain complications.
- *Foot or leg pain or numbness.* The most common cause of peripheral neuropathy is toxicity from stavudine (d4T, *Zerit*) or didanosine (ddI, *Videx*). Untreated HIV can do it, too. The treatment is with an ART regimen that doesn't include stavudine or didanosine (Question 45).
- *Seizures.* Anyone who has a seizure for the first time should go to an emergency room. After that, consult a neurologist, who will probably order an MRI scan of the brain with intravenous contrast to look for mass lesions.
- *Weakness, coordination problems, unsteady gait, or incontinence.* Depending on the location of the symptoms, you may need an MRI scan of the brain and/or spinal cord.

PART ELEVEN

Women's Issues, Pregnancy, and Children

How Is HIV infection different for women?

What if I want to get pregnant?

What if my child is positive?

More . . .

74. How Is HIV infection different for women?

For the most part, HIV infection in women is similar to HIV infection in men, but there are a few important differences. Some studies have shown that at the same CD4 counts, HIV-positive women have lower viral loads than HIV-positive men. This probably doesn't affect the decision of when to start treatment because that decision is mostly based on CD4 count and because the differences in viral load disappear with time.

Some studies have suggested that HIV-positive women die sooner than HIV-positive men, but that's because of delayed diagnosis. Women who are at greatest risk for HIV may have less access to health care. Those who are infected heterosexually may be less likely to get tested because they don't think they're at risk. Women who get diagnosed and treated for HIV infection live as long as men—longer in fact, since women generally tend outlive men.

Women respond well to ART. There are no HIV drugs that can't be used in women or that are specifically recommended for women.

Women respond well to ART. There are no HIV drugs that can't be used in women or that are specifically recommended for women. There are some gender-specific issues to be aware of, however. Nevirapine (*Viramune*) is more likely to cause liver toxicity in women than in men, and it's not recommended for women starting treatment with CD4 counts above 250, who are at greatest risk. Efavirenz (*Sustiva, Atripla*) can cause birth defects, so it shouldn't be taken by women who are sexually active with men and aren't using effective birth control. A number of PIs and NNRTIs may decrease the effectiveness of birth control pills, making them unreliable. Women taking drugs that interact with birth control pills should use an additional form of contraception, such as condoms or a diaphragm.

75. Does HIV cause gynecologic problems?

A number of common gynecologic problems can be more frequent or severe in HIV-positive women. *Candida* vaginitis (a vaginal infection cause by *Candida,* a common yeast) is a good example. More recurrent or serious candidiasis is sometimes the first sign of immunosuppression in HIV-positive women. Vaginitis can be treated with topical antifungal agents or with oral fluconazole.

Another vaginal infection that is more common in HIV-positive women is **bacterial vaginosis,** a bacterial infection that causes vaginal discharge. **Pelvic inflammatory disease (PID),** an infection of the uterus and fallopian tubes usually caused by sexually transmitted infections, can sometimes be more serious and may be more likely to require surgery in HIV-positive women.

As in men, genital herpes can become more severe or recur more frequently as the CD4 count falls. It causes painful genital ulcers that should be treated with anti-herpes medications. Genital herpes can increase the viral load and can make it easier to transmit HIV. Women who have frequent herpes outbreaks should take daily medication to prevent flares. HIV-positive women can also develop idiopathic genital ulcers—ulcers for which no cause is found. These are similar to aphthous ulcers in the mouth and esophagus (Questions 64 and 65). They usually occur in women with very low CD4 counts and are best treated with ART, along with the advice of a gynecologist who has is also an expert in treating HIV-positive women.

Human papillomavirus (HPV), discussed in Question 81, causes genital warts, cervical dysplasia, and cervical cancer.

> *Rose's comment:*
> *Before I was diagnosed I'd been battling yeast infections for 2 years, but the doctors didn't pick up on it. After I was diagnosed I learned that frequent or severe yeast infections can be a sign of HIV infection in women. I also had abnormal Pap smears caused by the HPV virus. HIV puts me at more risk for cervical problems than other women. Freezing didn't work, and I had to get a cone biopsy*

Bacterial vaginosis

A bacterial infection of the vagina that causes vaginal discharge.

Pelvic inflammatory disease (PID)

A serious infection of the uterus and fallopian tubes usually caused by sexually transmitted infections, especially gonorrhea and chlamydia.

where they cut the bad cells out of your cervix, just like coring an apple. It's important for HIV-positive women to get regular pelvic exams and Pap smears.

76. What if I want to get pregnant?

Pregnancy is a realistic option for HIV-positive women now that we can treat HIV effectively and prevent women from passing it to the baby. However, pregnancy should be carefully planned and closely monitored in HIV-positive women.

Pregnancy is a realistic option for HIV-positive women now that we can treat HIV effectively and prevent women passing it to the baby.

If you're not already on ART, don't need it urgently, and plan to get pregnant, you can consider waiting to start therapy until the second trimester. If you're already on ART, stay on it, but you may need to change your medications before trying to get pregnant.

ART is a *must* after the first trimester since transmission to the baby is extremely unlikely if the mother has an undetectable viral load at delivery. The only antiretroviral drug *known* to cause birth defects is efavirenz (*Sustiva, Atripla*). Women should *not* get pregnant if they're taking efavirenz or have taken it within the last month. Nevirapine (*Viramune*) is safe, but only in women with CD4 counts below 250. Once you're on nevirapine, it's safe to keep taking it after the CD4 count increases. Most pregnant women take a protease inhibitor. The most widely used PI in pregnancy is lopinavir/ritonavir (*Kaletra*), but other PIs can also be used. We have tended to use zidovudine/lamivudine (*Combivir*) as the NRTI part of the regimen in pregnant women because of its safety record. However, zidovudine can cause nausea, already a common symptom during pregnancy, so other NRTIs can be considered. Elective cesarean section is sometimes used to further reduce the risk of transmission to the baby, but it's only necessary if the viral load is detectable at the time of delivery.

If your partner is HIV-negative, you should conceive using artificial insemination to avoid infecting him, especially if your you're not on ART yet or have a detectable load. This can be done by a physician, or at home using the "turkey baster" approach, in which the partner's semen is squirted into the vagina using a turkey baster or syringe to avoid intercourse.

HIV-positive women who want to get pregnant should talk first to their provider and to an obstetrician-gynecologist who has HIV expertise. There are many other issues to discuss besides ART, including safe conception, planning the delivery, breastfeeding, and medical care for the baby, just to name a few.

Rose's comment:

My dream was always to have a big family, but I felt funny talking to medical providers about having more children because I was positive. My second child was infected because I didn't know I was positive during my pregnancy. My next child was negative because I took antiretroviral therapy, but I was scared to have more children, so I had my tubes tied. After I remarried, I realized I wanted a child with my husband. I started talking to my providers about pregnancy. Getting my tubes untied wasn't easy, but I finally found a fertility doctor who agreed to do it.

Then we had to talk about how to get pregnant without putting my HIV-negative husband at risk. We used the "turkey baster" method, which is artificial insemination done at home. I got pregnant within 3 months. Since I was taking antiretroviral therapy and had an undetectable viral load, I knew that there was very little risk of having another infected baby. I'm a great mom, and I plan on being around for my family for a long time.

77. How can I father a child with an HIV-negative woman?

Conception is more complicated when the male partner is positive because of the risk of infecting the woman. Having an undetectable viral load on ART is the most important thing you can do to prevent transmission, though there's still a very small chance of infection, since men can have virus in their semen even when it's undetectable in their blood.

Sperm washing

A technique in which sperm are separated from semen to lower the risk of HIV transmission to a woman during conception.

Sperm washing is a technique that involves separating sperm from semen to reduce the risk of transmission. To date there haven't been any reported cases of an HIV-negative woman becoming infected with this procedure, but sperm washing is only done at a few medical centers and is very expensive.

If you're going to try to conceive the "natural way," there are some things that can be done to reduce the risk. First, *don't* attempt this until the man's viral load is undetectable. Second, try to conceive only during the most fertile part of the woman's cycle, using home ovulation tests. Finally, the woman can consider using pre-exposure prophylaxis (PrEP) before attempting conception (Question 13). If you're contemplating this type of conception, get the advice of an expert first. It's also a good idea for both partners to be screened first for other sexually transmitted infections.

If both partners are infected, this is less of an issue. The HIV status of the father is irrelevant as far as the baby goes since an infant can only be infected by its mother.

78. What if my child is positive?

A thorough discussion of HIV in children is beyond the scope of this book, which is written for HIV-positive adults. Children and adolescents can be infected either through **perinatal transmission** (transmitted from the mother during late pregnancy, labor, or breastfeeding), or through the usual types of

Perinatal transmission

Transmission of HIV from mother to infant during late pregnancy, labor, or breastfeeding.

transmission (sex or drug use). Fortunately, mother-to-child transmission has become rare in the United States because of the routine testing of pregnant women and the use of ART during pregnancy.

Diagnosing babies is complicated because they carry the mother's HIV antibodies for up to 18 months, regardless of whether they're truly infected. Since the standard blood tests aren't helpful, **polymerase chain reaction (PCR)** testing of the blood is used to find the virus itself. Also, the CD4 counts that indicate immunosuppression in children under 5 are higher from those in older children and adults.

Without treatment, many HIV-positive babies can get sick within the first year of life. More often, they may do well initially for several years, not becoming ill until they enter pre-school or grade school. Untreated HIV-positive children may not gain weight or grow normally, and they may have neurologic problems that can cause delayed mental development, poor school performance, or cerebral palsy.

Treatment of children is similar to treatment of adults. However, not all drugs come in forms that kids can swallow, and there aren't as many studies on the treatment of children as there are for adults.

HIV-positive adolescents can be especially challenging...even more challenging than adolescents *without* HIV infection! Issues such as adherence, stigma, discrimination, disclosure, depression, substance abuse, and the prevention of further transmission can be especially daunting at this stage of life. HIV-positive adolescents need to be treated by providers who are experts both in HIV infection and adolescent medicine.

Rose's comment:
I found out I was infected when my daughter tested positive 2 months after she was born. It was only then that I

Women's Issues, Pregnancy, and Children

Diagnosing babies is complicated because they carry the mother's HIV antibodies for up to 18 months, regardless of whether they're truly infected.

Polymerase chain reaction (PCR)

A laboratory technique used to detect or quantify the DNA or RNA of an infectious organism for diagnostic purposes.

Without treatment, many HIV-positive babies can get sick within the first year of life.

learned that the man I was married to was at high risk. When I found out my daughter was infected, my own health care didn't matter; all I cared about was her. My doctors left me with the impression that she would die soon, which I refused to accept. I used myself as the guinea pig, trying medicines first before I let the doctors use them on her. In 1996, the new cocktails changed both our lives.

My CD4 count was 33 and my viral load was sky-high. All that changed on the cocktail, and my daughter responded beautifully as well. I knew then that we were both going to live. My daughter—the one who was going to die soon—is now 19 years old, has an undetectable viral load, and is starting her third year of college!

PART TWELVE

Coinfection

What if I also have hepatitis C?

What if I also have hepatitis B?

How do I prevent cervical and anal cancer?

More . . .

79. What if I also have hepatitis C?

Now that people aren't dying of AIDS as often, HCV has become an increasingly important cause of death among HIV-positive people.

"**Coinfection**" with both HIV and hepatitis C virus (HCV) is common, especially among injection drug users, since both viruses are easily passed from one person to another with shared needles or syringes. HCV can also be transmitted sexually, though not as easily as HIV and the hepatitis B virus (HBV). HCV is a common cause of severe liver disease, including **cirrhosis** (liver scarring) and **hepatocellular carcinoma (or hepatoma, or liver cancer)**. Now that people aren't dying of AIDS as often, HCV has become an increasingly important cause of death among HIV-positive people.

Untreated HIV infection can make hepatitis C get worse more rapidly. If you're coinfected with HIV and HCV, it's possible that ART will slow the progression of your hepatitis, though that's still somewhat controversial. You should get vaccinated against the hepatitis A and B viruses if you're not already immune, since those viruses can cause more severe disease in people with HCV infection. Finally, don't drink alcohol. Alcohol use, even in moderation, is a big risk factor for HCV progression.

Unlike HIV, hepatitis C can be cured, and it doesn't require life-long therapy. New drugs became available in 2011 that offer a great chance of cure, though not an easy one. HCV treatment is a lot more challenging than ART. For now, it generally means taking injectable **pegylated interferon**, which can cause fatigue, mood changes, and other side effects, plus oral medications that have their own challenges, both in terms of dosing frequency and side effects. As I write this, HCV treatment feels like HIV treatment did in 1996. We have exciting, promising new drugs, but they're difficult. New drugs are coming, and it will soon be possible to treat HCV without interferon. Talk to a specialist to find out whether you need to be treated now or whether you can afford to wait. This decision is mainly based on the amount of liver fibrosis you have, determined either by a **liver biopsy** or other measures of fibrosis.

Coinfection

The combination of two infections, such as HIV plus either hepatitis B virus or hepatitis C virus.

Cirrhosis

A form of permanent liver damage caused by alcoholism or chronic hepatitis.

Hepatocellular carcinoma (or hepatoma, or liver cancer)

A cancer of the liver that can be caused by alcoholism or chronic hepatitis.

Pegylated interferon

The preferred form of interferon, as it can be injected less frequently and has fewer side effects.

If your HCV is being treated by someone other than your HIV provider, make sure they communicate with each other. The new HCV drugs interact with antiretroviral medications. You may have to switch to a different ART regimen in order to be treated for HCV.

80. What if I also have hepatitis B?

It's not unusual to be infected with both HIV and the hepatitis B virus (HBV) since both are spread in the same way (sex and blood exposure). Most people who get infected with HBV clear the infection on their own, sometimes after getting sick with hepatitis and sometimes without ever knowing they were infected. However, others never clear the infection and go on to develop chronic HBV infection, which can lead to chronic hepatitis, cirrhosis, or liver cancer. HIV-positive people are more likely to develop chronic hepatitis B than HIV-negative people.

Everyone with HIV infection should be tested for HBV, and vice versa. A negative hepatitis B surface antigen (**HBsAg**) generally means you're not infected, though there are exceptions that can be diagnosed with an HBV DNA test. A positive surface antibody (**HBsAb**) means you've been exposed and are immune. If your antibody is negative, you should be vaccinated with a series of three shots. If your surface antibody and antigen are negative but your core antibody (HBcAb or anti-HBc IgG) is positive, you should still be checked for chronic hepatitis with an HBV DNA, and if that's negative, you should be vaccinated. You're more likely to respond to the vaccine if you wait until after you've responded to HIV therapy.

People who have both HIV and HBV should be treated for both infections at the same time, and with the same drugs. Trying to treat just one without causing resistance in other is too difficult, and involves taking less desirable medications. The easiest way to treat HIV/HBV coinfection is with an

Liver biopsy

The removal of a piece of the liver for diagnostic purposes, either with a needle inserted through the skin, or by a catheter inserted into a vein.

HBsAg

A blood test to diagnose acute or chronic hepatitis B.

HBsAb

A blood test to determine immunity to hepatitis B.

People who have both HIV and HBV should be treated for both infections at the same time.

Alpha-fetoprotein (AFP)

A blood test used to look for liver cancer.

Dysplasia

Abnormal development or growth of tissues, organs, or cells.

Stopping HBV drugs can lead to a dangerous flare of hepatitis.

Colposcopy

A procedure used to more closely examine the cervix for dysplasia due to human papillomavirus (HPV) infection in women who have had abnormal Pap smears.

Anal dysplasia

Abnormal cells in the anus caused by human papillomavirus (HPV). If left untreated, it can progress to anal cancer.

High resolution anoscopy (HRA)

A procedure used to more closely examine the lining of the anus for dysplasia due to human papillomavirus (HPV) infection in people who have had abnormal anal Pap smears.

ART combination that contains tenofovir and emtricitabine. For now, that means taking *Atripla*, *Complera*, or a combination of *Truvada* plus another drug. Lamivudine (3TC, *Epivir*, and contained in *Epzicom*, *Combivir*, *Trizivir*) is also active against both HIV and HBV. To avoid drug resistance, never take medications that treat both viruses unless they're being used in a complete ART.

Stopping HBV drugs can lead to a dangerous flare of hepatitis. People with chronic HBV infection should also get checked periodically for cirrhosis and liver cancer with a CT scan or ultrasound of the liver and the **alpha-fetoprotein (AFP)** blood test.

81. How do I prevent cervical and anal cancer?

Both cervical and anal cancer are caused by human papillomavirus (HPV), a sexually transmitted virus that first causes changes in the cells of the cervix and anus (**dysplasia**), which can later turn into cancer. HPV infection is common, and so is dysplasia. Fortunately, anal and cervical cancer are much less common and can be prevented.

The cervical Pap smear is a routine test for women to look for cervical dysplasia. HIV-positive women should get a Pap smear regularly—at least once a year. An abnormal Pap smear is evaluated by **colposcopy**, where abnormal areas can be looked at more closely and biopsied. High-grade lesions can then be treated with minor surgery.

Since **anal dysplasia** is also caused by HPV, involves similar cells, and can also progress to anal cancer, it makes sense to screen and treat anal dysplasia like we do cervical dysplasia. That's now possible using an anal Pap smear and **high resolution anoscopy (HRA)**, the anal equivalent of colposcopy. An anal Pap smear is a simple procedure: a wet swab is inserted in the anus and twisted around on its way out. But it doesn't make sense to do anal Pap smears unless there's someone available to follow-up abnormal results with anoscopy. Screening for anal dysplasia is not a standard recommendation yet, but many centers are doing it, especially in women and in gay and bisexual men. Straight men can have anal dysplasia too, even straight men who've never had sex with a man, so perhaps we should be doing this test in everybody.

There's now a vaccine to prevent HPV infection. It's not widely used in HIV-positive people yet, and many are already infected with HPV. This is a vaccine that's best used in children or adolescents before they become sexually active, but young HIV-positive people can consider vaccination, which is now approved for men and women less than 26 years old.

PART THIRTEEN

Mental Health and Substance Abuse

How do I know if I'm depressed?

What should I do if I'm depressed?

What are the risks of using drugs if I'm positive?

More . . .

82. How do I know if I'm depressed?

HIV-positive people who are depressed often assume they're just having a normal response to being positive. But depression, in the true medical sense of the word, is *never* "normal." People often describe themselves as being "depressed" when what they *really* mean is that they're sad, disappointed, angry, worried, or demoralized—perfectly normal responses to the bad things that happen to us in life. Depression, on the other hand, is not a normal response to life's misfortunes. Some people can be depressed for no apparent reason when everything's going well, while others go through difficult or unhappy lives without ever being depressed. While depression may be brought on by life events, it's probably more a result of brain chemistry than external circumstances.

People who are depressed feel sad, empty, hollow, hopeless, and isolated. Activities and people they once enjoyed no longer bring pleasure.

People who are depressed feel sad, empty, hollow, hopeless, and isolated. Activities and people they once enjoyed no longer bring pleasure. They may lose interest in sex, work, hobbies, friends, and family. They see no light at the end of the tunnel—the future looks bleak. They may have insomnia or they may sleep too much. They may lose their appetite for food or overeat. They may abuse drugs or alcohol in an attempt to feel better. Symptoms can include fatigue, weight loss (or gain), memory loss, and headache.

In contrast, people who are experiencing normal coping problems—dealing with an HIV diagnosis, for example—may feel sad, stressed, angry, or worried, but they understand that they'll get through it, and they can be "cheered up" or distracted by keeping busy or by being with people they enjoy.

If my description of depression rings true, talk to your medical provider immediately. Depression is a dangerous but highly treatable condition.

Rose's comment:
I knew I was depressed when I stopped wanting to get up or to clean my house. I lost interest in my children's

schools or being in the PTA. I isolated myself and was often tearful or angry. Everything was dark, and everything about me was dark. I stopped paying bills, and I didn't care about my appearance. Of course, I never should have waited until things got that bad. If it ever happened again, I'd know what to look for and would get help sooner.

> *Depression is a dangerous but highly treatable condition.*

83. What should I do if I'm depressed?

If you view depression as a normal emotion, a sign of weakness, or a character flaw, you're unlikely to get the help you need. Think of depression as though it were pneumonia. You *might* get better on your own, but it won't be pleasant. It could take a long time, and it *could* even kill you. With treatment, things can get better fast.

The best way to treat depression is to take **antidepressants**—drugs that restore the balance of chemicals in your brain that are out of balance when you're depressed. There are many antidepressants available. They all work to treat depression but have different side effects. Some antidepressants are sedating and can be helpful for people with insomnia. Others can perk you up if you're fatigued or sleeping too much. Some antidepressants can cause sexual side effects, especially delayed orgasm. Most antidepressants also help control anxiety and obsessive thoughts.

Antidepressants
Drugs used to treat depression.

When you take an antidepressant, don't expect sudden or dramatic changes. It can take 2 to 4 weeks before you start to notice a difference in how you're feeling. The point isn't to change your personality or to make you ecstatically happy. The point of antidepressants is to help make you feel like yourself again. Antidepressants won't change the circumstances of your life, but they can help you cope with those circumstances. They're not habit forming—they can be tapered and stopped when you no longer need them. If you don't tolerate the first drug you try, don't give up. Switch to a drug with a different side effect profile.

> *The best way to treat depression is to take antidepressants—drugs that restore the balance of chemicals in your brain that are out of balance when you're depressed.*

Counseling and psychotherapy are not a substitute for medications because in the depths of depression, talking doesn't do much good. Talk therapy becomes useful as you start to get better—it helps you return to life, to deal with issues that might have contributed to your depression, and to keep you healthy after you get better. Psychotherapy is also great for people who aren't depressed but are having problems coping with life circumstances.

Rose's comment:
I was afraid to talk about my depression to Joel (my provider) because back then he was still one of those "white coat guys" that I didn't trust. But I started talking to other people in the waiting room at the clinic, and I realized I wasn't alone—other people had been through this before. When I finally talked to Joel about my depression, he started me on an antidepressant. I slowly began to feel better, and then I realized just how bad I'd let things get. It took about 30 days before I got my energy back and was myself again. The experience also taught me that I could talk to Joel about these things and that he would listen and care. It's very important to have a provider you can talk to.

84. What are the risks of using drugs if I'm positive?

HIV-positive people often assume that drug use is bad for them because it lowers their CD4 count and increases their viral load, but that's not the reason to stay away from drugs. (I wish we could say that "good, clean living" would keep HIV under control, but life isn't fair, and the virus doesn't care what you do.) Still, there are plenty of other great reasons to stay away from drugs.

First, there are the medical dangers of the drugs themselves. Cocaine causes heart attacks and mental illness. Heroin injection can lead to serious infections of the heart valves, bones, and joints. Methamphetamine can destroy your teeth, your brain, your relationships, your career, and your life. All three are addictive. It's hard to come up with too many dire warnings about the dangers of marijuana, but even its advocates admit that regular use can make you dumb and lazy, and there's now some evidence that it could increase the risk of mental illness later in life. There is evidence that *Aspergillus*, a fungus that can cause dangerous infections in people with very low CD4 counts, can live in marijuana leaves and can be inhaled. (If you smoke dope and have a low CD4 count, some recommend microwaving the joint to kill the fungus. Please don't ask me which setting to use or for how long—those studies will never be done!)

Second, drugs can also interact with your HIV medications. Drug companies don't typically study interactions between their drugs and illegal substances. But there is evidence that people have been harmed by taking "club drugs," such as MDMA (Ecstasy) and ketamine, along with antiretrovirals.

Drug use can increase your risk of getting other infections or of spreading HIV to others. Being high lowers your inhibitions and clouds your judgment, allowing you to take risks that you wouldn't otherwise take, putting you at risk for sexually transmitted diseases, including syphilis (Question 88). Injection is especially risky, since it can spread HIV, hepatitis C, and other bloodborne infections.

Finally, studies show that active drug users are less likely to take ART correctly, putting them at risk of drug resistance and loss of treatment options. If you've got a drug problem, get treatment before you start ART. Don't wait until you've messed up and developed drug resistance.

Ultimately, the best reason to stay away from drugs is to keep yourself physically and mentally healthy so you'll have the upper hand against HIV infection.

Aspergillus
A fungus that causes aspergillosis, a potentially serious infection involving the lungs that can occur in people with very advanced HIV disease.

Drug use can increase your risk of getting other infections or of spreading HIV to others.

If you've got a drug problem, get treatment before you start ART.

PART FOURTEEN

Relationships, Sexuality, and Prevention

How and when should I disclose my
HIV status to partners?

How can I have safe sex?

What should I know about
sexually transmitted infections?

More . . .

85. How and when should I disclose my HIV status to partners?

Being HIV-positive doesn't mean you can't have intimate relationships or sex, but it does complicate things since you have to deal with revealing your HIV status to partners and protecting those who are negative from becoming infected.

The issue of disclosure can be a thorny one. Some argue that disclosure isn't necessary if you're practicing safe sex. They point out that everyone knows the risks and should be protecting themselves, regardless of what their partners say—or don't say—about their status. There are also situations where disclosure is unrealistic. Anonymous sex taking place in a sex club or dark alley rarely involves a "How do you do," much less a detailed exchange of medical information. Then again, someone having sex in that environment should assume a high level of risk and take the appropriate precautions.

Disclosure becomes especially important when you're dating or starting a new relationship. Some people deal with this by dating only HIV-positive partners. That simplifies things, but it's not possible for everyone. Disclosing your status to a negative partner can be a deal breaker, resulting not only in rejection but the risk that your new "ex" may share your information with others. For that reason, many choose to wait until there's mutual affection, trust, and a sense that the relationship is going somewhere.

The problem is that the longer you wait, the more likely your new partner will feel betrayed when you finally disclose your status, especially if the relationship has already become sexual. If you're positive and your goal is to be in a relationship, you may have to take things slower than we're used to these days. Get to know and trust your partner first, talk about your HIV status next, and *then* have sex. If this process takes a while, that's OK. Remember—in Jane Austen's day, couples didn't even use first names until the engagement was announced!

Rose's comment:
Disclosing your status isn't easy, especially to a partner.
I sat him down and just blurted out that I was positive.
He asked me how it happened, and I explained that I'd
been infected by my first husband. I don't know which
scared him more, my HIV or the fact that my tubes were
tied, but he ran. I thought I'd never see him again. But
he was back 2 weeks later. He said he wanted to learn
more, and I started educating him about HIV. We talked
about condom use, and I told him condoms should be
mandatory in any relationship because of HIV and other
sexually transmitted infection. We built our relationship
from there, and now we've been married for over 8 years.

86. How can I have safe sex?

There is no sexual activity that is guaranteed to transmit HIV infection, and there's at least *some* risk involved in most activities—at least the most popular ones. I can't give you odds or percentages, since the risk depends not only on what you're doing, but on how you're doing it and your viral load. The risk is dramatically reduced if the viral load is undetectable. We can't say it's zero, since it's possible to have detectable virus in semen or vaginal fluid even when it's undetectable in blood. Still, being on effective ART is probably the most effective way to prevent transmission if you're going to have sex. Here are some general comments about the "riskiness" of the more common sexual activities.

- *Anal and vaginal intercourse.* If the positive partner is "on top," this is a high-risk activity without a condom. An intact condom reduces the risk dramatically if it doesn't break. The risk is lower if the positive partner is on the bottom. That's because the lining of the anus and vagina is made of **mucosal cells,** which can be infected, whereas the penis is almost completely covered by skin, which can't. However, a man can still get infected from insertive intercourse. The risk is higher if he's uncircumcised or has

Mucosal cells

Cells that line the internal organs and body orifices, such as the mouth, nostrils, anus, and genital area.

herpes, syphilis, or other open sores on his penis. The risk of spreading both HIV and the hepatitis C virus increases if there's bleeding during sex.

- *Oral sex.* HIV can be transmitted by getting a positive person's preseminal fluid ("pre-cum"), semen ("cum"), vaginal fluid, or menstrual blood in the mouth. (It's not a question of swallowing.) The risk is higher if the gums are in bad shape. If the positive partner is the one "going down" on the negative partner, there's essentially no risk of HIV transmission, though other STIs can be spread that way.
- *Oral-anal sex ("rimming").* This is not an easy way to spread HIV, but the person doing the rimming could get hepatitis A or a bacterial or parasitic gastrointestinal infection.
- *Mutual masturbation.* This is very safe as long as you don't have open cuts or sores on the hands and keep things out of the mouth and eyes.
- *"Water sports."* Urine is a safe bodily fluid.
- *Kissing, hugging, cuddling, massage.* All safe.

87. What if my partner is negative?

Let's assume that disclosure is out of the way (Question 85). You're positive and your negative partner knows it. What next?

It's your responsibility to make sure you never infect *anyone*, including your negative partner. "This infection stops with me" are words to live by. Of course, HIV-negative adults should be aware of the risks and should be protecting themselves as well. Unfortunately, that approach hasn't been working, and the epidemic continues to grow. Prevention experts are now changing the prevention message to focus on those who are positive—people who know better than anyone how important it is to prevent transmission and who must bear most of the responsibility for not spreading the infection.

Uninfected people sometimes make crazy choices and stupid decisions. Some may seem perfectly willing to put themselves at risk of infection. It's the moral obligation of the positive partner not to cooperate with that kind of self-destructive behavior, to ensure that their HIV is never transmitted. "Every man for himself" is not a philosophy that promotes a world we want to live in. We live in a community and should watch out for each other.

That being said, risk is relative. Once the clothes come off, it's not usually a choice between high-risk and no-risk activities, but between high-risk and lower-risk. For more on the relative risk of various sexual activities, see Question 86.

88. What if both my partner and I are positive?

Being with a positive partner eliminates concerns about new HIV transmission, but there are still reasons to consider safe sex, including avoidance of other sexually transmitted infections (Question 89) and **superinfection**. We know that HIV-positive people can be superinfected with additional strains of virus. There have been some well-documented cases, which also explains why there are **recombinant strains** of HIV in the world (viruses that are combinations of two or more **subtypes**). Superinfection can cause a rise in viral load and a drop in CD4 count, similar to what happens with initial infection. You could also become superinfected with a drug-resistant strain of virus, especially if you were taking drugs that your partner's virus was resistant to.

Proving superinfection requires the kind of testing that isn't readily available through commercial labs, so we don't know how often it occurs. It's probably not common, and there's evidence that it happens mostly to people who have been recently infected—within a few years—but not in those with longstanding infection.

Superinfection can cause a rise in viral load and a drop in CD4 count, similar to what happens with initial infection.

Superinfection

Reinfection with a new strain of HIV in someone who has already been infected.

Recombinant strains

Strains of HIV that are combinations of two or more other strains.

Sub-types

In the case of HIV, groups of related viruses, also called "clades" or "sub-clades."

Relationships, Sexuality, and Prevention

When talking to my positive patients about sex with other positive partners, I recommend that they use condoms with casual partners, mainly to prevent sexually transmitted infections. In steady relationships, the decision to abandon condoms will depend on how long each partner has been infected, whether they're monogamous, their viral loads, whether either partner has resistant virus, whether or not they're likely to be infected with the same strain (did one get infected by the other?), and whether there are other transmittable infections to consider, such as hepatitis C virus.

89. What should I know about sexually transmitted infections?

Becoming positive doesn't mean you can stop worrying about sexually transmitted infections (STIs). You've got the Big One, but there are others to be avoided. Safe sex is still the way to go.

Syphilis can be worse in people with HIV infection. It can progress more rapidly if it's not treated. It's more likely to infect the nervous system, and can affect your vision and hearing. The blood tests we use to monitor your response to syphilis treatment can be harder to interpret and can take longer to become negative than in HIV-negative people. If you're HIV-positive, you should be checked for syphilis, and the test should be repeated at least once a year if you're sexually active.

Gonorrhea and chlamydia are common infections that can infect the urethra of the penis, the cervix, the anus, and the throat. Gonorrhea has become resistant to standard oral antibiotics and must now be treated with an injection. HIV-positive men should be checked for gonorrhea and chlamydia with a urine test and sometimes with anal and/or throat swabs; women should be tested at the time of their routine pelvic exam. A different type of chlamydial infection, **lymphogranuloma venereum (LGV)** is now being reported causing anal and rectal infections (**proctitis**) in gay men.

Becoming positive doesn't mean you can stop worrying about sexually transmitted infections.

Lymphogranuloma venereum (LGV)

A sexually transmitted infection caused by *Chlamydia*.

Proctitis

Infection or inflammation of the rectum.

Genital herpes, usually caused by herpes simplex virus type 2 (HSV-2), causes painful blisters and shallow ulcers on the genitals, around the anus, or on the skin. The infection persists for life and can recur, especially in people with low CD4 counts. ART can help, but outbreaks should be treated with an anti-herpes medication, such as acyclovir, famciclovir, or valacyclovir. If you're having frequent outbreaks, you should take one of those medications daily, which not only prevents herpes flares, but may help lower your HIV viral load and the risk of herpes (and possibly HIV) transmission. HSV-1 usually causes cold sores on the lips (herpes labialis); it isn't usually a recurring problem "below the waist."

Human papillomavirus (HPV) infection is discussed in Question 81. There are other STIs that I haven't discussed but that are also best avoided.

Relationships, Sexuality, and Prevention

PART FIFTEEN

Living With HIV Infection

What foods and water are safe?

Should I take vitamins or supplements?

Can I travel abroad?

More . . .

90. What foods and water are safe?

There are few foods you should *avoid* eating because of HIV infection, but there are some guidelines to follow, especially if your CD4 count is low. Avoid undercooked meat, especially if your *Toxoplasma* antibody is negative (Question 56). Avoid raw eggs, undercooked poultry, unpasteurized milk or fruit juices, and raw sprouts. Hard cheeses (like cheddar) are safer than soft cheeses (like brie, feta, Camembert, or Mexican cheeses), which may contain *Listeria,* a bacterium that can cause meningitis (though not often). Avoiding raw shellfish is a good idea, but if you can't resist a raw oyster, make sure you're immune to hepatitis A (Question 26). Some doctors recommend avoiding sushi, but that seems cruel and extreme to me, and the bugs you can get from sushi aren't much worse if you're HIV-positive. Be careful not to "cross-contaminate" food when you're preparing it. For good food safety tips, check out http://www.foodsafety.gov/.

What *should* you eat? Healthy food, preferably *real* food: food that you or someone else cooks from original, pronounceable ingredients. Eat fresh fruits and vegetables—with every meal, every day. If you eat meat, don't eat it all the time; eat more poultry and fish. Your starches should be brown, not white; the white, refined ones just get turned into sugar. And speaking of sugar, think of dessert as a special treat, not a course. To gain weight, eat more. To lose weight, eat less. Break the rules once in awhile, but not too often. When you break the rules, do it without guilt.

Finally, remember that eating is not a form of medical therapy but one of life's great pleasures. Take your time and enjoy it!

What about water? For most HIV-positive people, tap water is perfectly safe. If you're not familiar with the term "tap water," it refers to a plentiful, delicious beverage that people used to drink directly from faucets and drinking fountains without charge, but that has been replaced by an expensive, bottled version that I call "tap water from a city you don't live in." How millions of gullible Americans were duped into voluntarily handing over large amounts of money for something that is still free is a great mystery, but it happened—the discarded plastic evidence of it is everywhere.

The best reasons to pay for water are if your tap water tastes bad, is known to be of bad quality, or if you like it fizzy. Otherwise, tap water is fine for most HIV-positive people. However, if your CD4 count is below 100, be aware of the risk of cryptosporidiosis. *Cryptosporidium* is a parasite that can be passed from person to person or ingested in contaminated water. Tap water is usually safe, but there have been occasional outbreaks when the water supply becomes contaminated. You can protect yourself by filtering tap water through a 100 micron filter. Bottled water is OK, too, but only if the company filters it in the same way.

Cryptosporidium is a parasite that can be passed from person to person or ingested in contaminated water.

91. Should I take vitamins or supplements?

If you've just read the previous answer, you can probably guess how I'm going to answer this one. A healthy diet should provide you with all the nutrients you need. If your diet is poor, then taking a multivitamin is a good idea. Vitamin supplements are good for you if you're vitamin deficient, but there's little evidence that they help you if you're already eating well. In fact, studies are finding that they can sometimes hurt you. A standard multivitamin is harmless and cheap, but I hate to see people spending lots of their hard-earned cash on the latest supplement touted on the web or at the health food store, money they could be spending on eating really good food. (By the way, if you're going to take vitamins, don't spend a lot of money. Compare ingredients and buy the cheap, generic stuff.)

Vitamin D and calcium supplements are good for people with osteopenia (thin bones, Question 50). Vitamin D deficiency is a hot topic these days. It's very common in both HIV-negative and HIV-positive people, and may be worse if you're taking efavirenz (*Sustiva, Atripla*), so taking a daily supplement isn't a bad idea.

I don't want to come across as a nutritional nihilist. I definitely believe in nutrition; I just think that it's best achieved by eating well.

92. Can I still drink alcohol?

The answer depends on whether it would have been OK for you to drink if you were HIV-negative. HIV infection itself has little to do with it. First, let's talk about who should *not* drink.

1. People with chronic hepatitis B or C shouldn't drink because it can make the hepatitis worse and increase the risk of cirrhosis (see Questions 78 and 79).
2. Alcoholics shouldn't drink because few are capable of drinking in moderation. Excessive alcohol consumption is bad for just about every organ in your body. It is especially bad for your liver, which can already be stressed by some of the medication we use to treat HIV infection. There are other conditions that can be caused by both alcohol abuse and by either HIV infection or ART, including neuropathy, dementia, blood disorders, heart problems, and pancreatitis, just to name a few. Why increase your risk? Finally, people who are drunk aren't good at taking medications, and we've already talked about what happens when you don't take your medications (Question 29). If you're not sure whether you're an alcoholic, there's a good chance you are. If alcohol has repeatedly caused problems with your work, relationships or criminal or driving record, if you can't control your drinking, if other people think you drink too much, if you feel guilty or lie about your drinking, if you wake up hung over or shaky until you get an eye-opener, then you've got a problem, one that needs to be addressed *before* you start HIV therapy.

If you can drink in moderation and have no medical reason to avoid alcohol, then drinking is OK with HIV and with HIV medications. Keep it down to a maximum of two drinks per day: two glasses of wine, two beers, or two ounces of hard liquor. (And if you don't drink all week, that doesn't mean you can have 14 drinks on Friday night!)

93. Can I travel abroad?

Yes, but there are a few things to consider, especially if you're going to a developing country where there are bugs you wouldn't normally come in contact with. If your CD4 count is over 200, then the risk is about the same as it would be for anyone else. But if your count is low, especially less than 50, then you might reconsider your destination or wait until your count is higher.

The CDC web site (www.cdc.gov/travel/) has excellent country-specific information about precautions and vaccinations. HIV-positive people should generally avoid vaccines that contain live viruses or bacteria. This is especially true for oral **typhoid vaccine** (get the injectable vaccine instead). If **yellow fever** vaccine is required and your CD4 count is low, you could consider going somewhere else. Getting the vaccine is reasonable if you have a high CD4 count and there's a definite risk of yellow fever. Make sure you've had a tetanus booster in the last 10 years and have been vaccinated against hepatitis A and B if you're not already immune (Question 25). Take the usual precautions to avoid travelers' diarrhea, and talk to your doctor about bringing an antibiotic along to treat it if it happens.

No matter where you're going, make sure you have enough meds for the entire trip and then some—plan ahead for cancelled or delayed flights. Bring the original bottles to avoid problems at the airport, and carry them on the plane rather than checking them in your luggage.

If you can drink in moderation and have no medical reason to avoid alcohol, then drinking is OK with HIV and with HIV medications.

Typhoid vaccine

A vaccine to prevent typhoid fever, a bacterial infection of the blood caused by *Salmonella typhi*, sometimes acquired by travelers to developing countries.

HIV-positive people should generally avoid vaccines that contain live viruses or bacteria.

Yellow fever

A serious disease caused by yellow fever virus, which is transmitted by mosquitoes and sometimes acquired by travelers to parts of Africa or Latin America.

Living With HIV Infection

Finally, consider taking the names of some HIV doctors or clinics in the areas you're traveling to, especially if your medical condition is complex or if you'll be away for a long time.

Bon voyage!

94. Can I keep my pets?

Don't go drowning Kitty in the river just because you're HIV-positive! You can still have pets if you follow a few simple precautions. If possible, stay away from very young animals (less than 6 months old), and avoid contact with sick animals. Pets with diarrhea should get checked for bugs in their feces that could be passed on to you. Wash your hands well after handling your pets and before eating.

Cats can carry *Toxoplasma gondii,* the parasite that causes toxoplasmosis (Question 56), which you get it from eating cat poop. "But I don't eat cat poop!" you protest. These things can happen, usually if you've been changing a litter box and get it on your hands and then in your mouth. Assuming you're not already infected (find out whether you have a positive *Toxoplasma* antibody), the best solution is to get someone else to change the litter box. If you and Kitty live alone together, then wear gloves, wash your hands, and change the box every day because it's harder to get toxo from fresh poop. Indoor kitties are safer than the outdoor prowlers. Take the same precautions with gardening, too.

Peliosis hepatis

An uncommon liver infection caused by *Bartonella.*

Cats can also transmit *Bartonella,* the bacterium that causes cat-scratch disease in children as well as bacillary angiomatosis (a skin disease) and **peliosis hepatis** (an infection of the liver) in HIV-positive people. Older cats are safer than young ones. Don't play rough with Kitty. Fortunately these are uncommon, treatable conditions—not a justification for de-clawing as a preventative measure. Sorry, but you can't use your HIV status as an excuse to save your sofa!

Reptiles, chicks, and ducklings can carry *Salmonella,* a bacterium that causes diarrhea and other problems, especially in HIV-positive people. Wash well after handling Mr. Lizard or consider trading him in for a different animal. There have also been reports of *Salmonella* in common pet treats so don't share them with your animals.

What about dogs? I have nothing bad to say about dogs.

95. Can I still exercise?

You can and you should. Mainly because it's a healthy way to live, and it's important to maintain your overall health if you're HIV-positive. But there are some reasons to exercise that are specific to HIV as well.

1. Some antiretroviral drugs can cause fat accumulation, insulin resistance, and elevations in cholesterol and triglycerides (Questions 43 and 46), which in turn can increase the risk of heart disease. Aerobic exercise helps to reverse all of those conditions.

2. Although we don't know the cause, we're seeing loss of bone density in people with HIV infection (Question 50). Exercise, especially resistance exercise, can help to maintain bone density.

3. Some of the older antiretroviral drugs cause lipoatrophy (fat loss) involving the legs, arms, and buttocks (Question 46). Resistance training can increase the muscle mass in these areas, which can help to compensate for the loss in fat. (Note that vigorous aerobic exercise, while great for fat accumulation, may make lipoatrophy worse...there's no justice!)

4. HIV-positive people are at greater risk for depression. Exercise is a great natural antidepressant.

If you're not used to exercising, start slow. Walk more. Take the stairs. Park in the far corner of the lot. If you're a fair weather walker, join a gym. Don't do the same type of exercise each day, but mix it up so you don't get bored. Exercise with a friend, or listen to music or a recorded book. A slug-like existence may be more likely to kill you than HIV, so don't be a slug!

96. What are advance directives?

Everybody dies. Whether you have HIV, some other chronic disease, or are the picture of health, you will someday take your last breath. Before we had effective treatment for HIV disease, an untimely death from AIDS was almost a certainty. In those days, I spent a lot of time talking to my patients about death and dying and helping them to make end-of-life decisions. Today, we spend more time talking about life, old age, and retirement, but I still encourage my patients (and friends and family members) to make plans and discuss their wishes about death and dying with the people who matter. The best time to think about these things is when you're healthy and have no immediate plans to leave this earth.

What kind of medical care would you want if you were sick and unable to make decisions for yourself? Would you want life-sustaining measures—to be resuscitated with **CPR** or to be put on a breathing machine in the intensive care unit—if the chances of recovery were low? Would you want any treatment at all, including artificial feeding, if you had a terminal illness? Who would you choose to make medical decisions for you?

If you know the answers to these questions, you need **advance directives**—legal documents that make your wishes known to others in case you can't speak for yourself. A **Living Will** is a legal document that lets you spell out the medical treatments and life-sustaining measures you would want or not want if you were unable to make those decisions for yourself. A Living Will is important, but it's not enough because it

CPR

Cardiopulmonary resuscitation. Procedures used to try to revive someone whose heart has stopped and/or has stopped breathing.

Advance directives

Legal documents that allow you to make decisions about end-of-life care ahead of time.

Living Will

A legal document that allows you to state which medical procedures and life-sustaining measures you would want if you were no longer able to make decisions for yourself.

doesn't cover every decision that might need to be made. It's also important to choose the person who would make medical decisions for you if you couldn't make them for yourself. If that person is your legally recognized spouse, then you're covered, because your spouse is automatically your next of kin. But if you want decisions to be made by an unmarried partner, a married partner not recognized as your spouse by our backward federal government, a friend, or a different family member, then you need to appoint that person using a **Durable Power of Attorney for Health Care,** a legal document that trumps next of kin rules. This document also allows your partner or friend to visit you in the hospital if visitation is otherwise limited to immediate family members. The person you appoint should be aware of your wishes in advance—including what's in your Living Will—and should agree to act in accordance with those wishes.

Everyone should have these documents. You don't need a lawyer—the forms are available online and in most clinics and hospitals. Give a copy to your provider and to the person you've named as your decision maker.

You should also have a will, especially if you want your belongings to go to someone other than your immediate family members. Whether you'll need a lawyer to draw up a will depends on how complex your finances and your wishes are. Simple wills can be drafted using software programs.

No one likes to think or talk about dying, but the consequences of not having advance directives can be tragic. Make your wishes known, and make them count!

Living With HIV Infection

Durable Power of Attorney for Health Care

A legal document that allows you to authorize someone else to make medical decisions on your behalf if you loose the ability to make decisions for yourself.

Questions

Those Who Still

Have Questions

What about the theory that HIV doesn't cause
AIDS?

Isn't it true that drug companies are withholding the
cure to make money?

What's the state of the global epidemic?

More . . .

. What about the theory that HIV doesn't cause AIDS?

In the early years of the AIDS epidemic, shortly after the discovery of HIV, a few scientists argued that AIDS was not caused by HIV infection. They proposed a number of alternative explanations, suggesting that AIDS was caused by drug abuse and zidovudine (in the developed world) and malnutrition (in the developing world). These scientists argued that **Koch's postulates** had not been fulfilled and warned that antiretroviral therapy, rather than saving lives, was prematurely ending them.

Koch's postulates

The four criteria needed to prove that a microbe or organism is the cause of a disease. (See Glossary for details.)

If their hypothesis was far-fetched in the late-80s, it's complete lunacy today. Koch's postulates have been fulfilled many times over. We now have a solid and ever growing understanding of how HIV infects human cells, damages the immune system, and causes AIDS. The life-saving effects of antiretroviral therapy have been well-established by countless clinical trials, large observational studies, and data from large populations. It was no accident that the death rate from AIDS declined by 50% in the year after HAART was introduced!

The so-called "scientists" who cling to their discredited hypotheses have forgotten one of the fundamental principles of science. You have to be able to admit that you might be wrong. Their dwindling followers (most have either died prematurely or have come to their senses and started therapy) now treat "HIV denialism" more as a cult than as a scientific hypothesis. These nut-jobs would be amusing if it weren't for their modest influence. They affected the policies of the South African government for many years, resulting in years of preventable deaths and new infections, and they have influenced gullible people not to get treated for a fatal disease. They have a lot to atone for.

98. Isn't it true that drug companies are withholding the cure to make money?

This is a popular point of view among conspiracy theorists and those with contempt for drug companies, but a little rational thought should put this myth to rest.

1. It's no surprise that we haven't yet cured HIV infection. The difficulty of finding a cure is discussed in Question 42.

2. People who develop therapies at drug companies are scientists. They're motivated by the things that motivate scientists everywhere else: publication in prestigious journals, the respect of their colleagues, Nobel Prizes, TV interviews, getting funding to do more research; and the knowledge that their work has made a difference to humankind. No scientist who discovers the cure for AIDS is going to keep quiet about it, even if ordered to do so by an evil, profit-hungry CEO!

3. Drug companies are competitive. If they're onto something big, they know their competitors can't be far behind. Being the *second* company to come up with The Cure won't be nearly important as being the first. If a company had a cure, you'd have heard about it!

4. A cure for AIDS would be highly profitable. Sure, there's profit in lifetime therapy, too, but it's shared among multiple competing drug companies and doesn't last forever. Drugs go off patent and get replaced by generics; they fall out of favor as they're replaced by newer and better agents. A cure is likely to be expensive and would result in an instant monopoly for the company that discovered it.

5. *Most* conspiracy theories are wrong.

99. How do we know HIV wasn't created in a lab?

This popular conspiracy theory gives way too much credit to the science of bygone generations. HIV first infected humans in the first half of the twentieth century. We have proof of human infection dating back to the '50s, and it probably became a human disease several decades before that. The idea that such a complex virus could be created by scientists today is far-fetched enough, but to think that it could have been invented 80 years ago is preposterous.

Throughout history, there have been infamous examples of abuse of the human race by science and medicine, but the deliberate creation of the HIV epidemic is not one of them.

Few of those who believe in this theory think it was just an innocent scientific experiment gone wrong. Instead, they think it was part of a well-orchestrated plot to rid the country—or the world—of its "undesirable" elements: gay men, injection drug users, or minorities...take your pick. But in the first half of the last century, we were too busy worrying about poverty (the '30s), the war ('40s), and communists (the '50s) to waste time trying to figure out how to wipe out gay men and drug users, who were barely on the radar screens of anyone except *other* gay men and drug users.

The fact that the HIV epidemic didn't originate in the developed world (where, as we know, all the evil scientists live) doesn't fit well with this theory either. Since the epidemic began in Africa, you'd have to propose that someone was trying to wipe out all Africans, a strategy that would not have been appreciated by the colonial powers who relied on them for labor and income.

Finally, it's inconceivable that the inventor of such a virus could have planned an epidemic that would target specific groups of people. Its spread among gay men, drug users, and minorities was accidental, and of course it didn't stay confined to those groups. Throughout history, there have been infamous examples of abuse of the human race by science and medicine, but the deliberate creation of the HIV epidemic is not one of them.

100. What's the state of the global epidemic?

I've been fairly upbeat in this book, talking about HIV infection as the chronic, manageable disease that it's become. That's because if you're reading this book, you probably live in a place where treatment is available and affordable. However, it's harder to be optimistic about the state of the global epidemic. More than 25 million people have died of AIDS, and more than 33 million are now living with HIV infection, most of them in developing countries. There are 2.6 million new cases of HIV every year, and AIDS kills over 2 million people every year. AIDS has wiped out hard-earned economic and healthcare gains in many developing countries, drastically reducing life expectancy and creating millions of orphans, whose prognosis is grim regardless of their HIV status. The epidemic threatens to cause economic, social, and civil collapse in countries where large proportions of the population—including the leaders, teachers, doctors, and civil servants—are infected and dying.

The news hasn't been *all* bad. The developed world finally recognized that it couldn't go on ignoring the devastation in the developing world, and money began flowing from the government, private, and philanthropic sectors began to provide life-saving treatment for people throughout the world, or at least in those countries where there was a political will to deal with the AIDS epidemic. Generic drugs made treatment more affordable.

But the global financial crisis now threatens the progress we've made. The flow of funds has slowed and could dry up altogether. In addition, the treatment being offered in most of the world would be considered second class by our standards. Viral load and resistance testing are rarely used, and fewer drugs are available, so options are limited if the first regimen fails. Most importantly, the number of new infections is far higher than the number of people being started on treatment—despite our progress, we fall further behind each year.

I can't begin to do justice to these issues here in Question 100. My hope is that HIV-positive people who read this will see themselves as part of a larger global community, one in which there are enormous inequities but great promise and hope. Our planet hasn't faced such a crisis in its history. How we confront this crisis will determine our future and what those who live in the future say about us. We have the resources, the intelligence, and the creativity to solve this problem. . .all we need is the will and the right sense of priorities.

Additional Resources

This book is by no means comprehensive. If you've read it cover to cover, you've just dipped your toe in the water. There are many good sources of information for HIV-positive people, much of it on the Internet. The following is just a partial list.

Web Sites

- *AIDS.gov.* Basic information on HIV and on U.S. government strategy and programs. http://aids.gov/.
- *AIDSInfo.* A site of the U.S. Department of Health and Human Services (DHHS), where you can find the latest treatment guidelines, drug information, and news about clinical trials. www.aidsinfo.nih.gov/.
- *AIDS Infonet.* A project of the New Mexico AIDS Education and Training Center that provides information on HIV treatment and prevention in multiple languages. http://www.aidsinfonet.org/.
- *AIDSmeds.com.* A good source of information about HIV treatment. http://www.aidsmeds.com/.
- *AIDS Portal.* HIV & AIDS and health related information with emphasis on global issues. Includes on-line forums. http://www.aidsportal.org/web/guest/home.
- *AIDS Teatment* News. A newsletter for HIV-positive people. www.aidsnews.org/.
- *American Academy of HIV Medicine.* You can find information about HIV providers in your area. www.aahivm .org.
- *AmfAR (American Foundation for AIDS Research).* Provides information on HIV, including research developments. http://www.amfar.org/.
- *Avert.org.* Domestic and international HIV information, news and stories. http://www.avert.org/#
- *BETA (Bulletin of Experimental Treatments for AIDS).* A bulletin published by the San Francisco AIDS Foundation covering new developments in HIV therapy. www.sfaf.org/beta/.

- *The Body.* A patient-oriented site that provides updated information, coverage of new scientific findings, and answers to users' questions. www.thebody.com.
- *CDC National Center for HIV/AIDS, Viral Hepatitis, STD, and TB Prevention.* CDC website with basic HIV information and data on U.S. epidemic. http://www .cdc.gov/nchhstp/.
- *Clinical Trials.gov.* A source of up-to-date information about federally and privately supported clinical research studies, including trials of HIV therapies. www.clinical trials.gov.
- *GMHC (Gay Men's Health Crisis).* A patient-oriented web site that provides basic HIV information and news. www.gmhc.org/.
- *HIVandHepatitis.com.* Scientific updates. http://www .hivandhepatitis.com/.
- *HIV Insight.* HIV information from the University of California, San Francisco. www.hivinsight.org/.
- *NATAP (National AIDS Treatment Advocacy Project).* Excellent source of information on new scientific data on HIV and hepatitis C, including studies presented at scientific conferences. http://www.natap.org/.
- *New York State Department of Health AIDS Institute.* Provides general information about HIV/AIDS. http:// www.health.state.ny.us/diseases/aids/.
- *POZ.* An online and print magazine for HIV-positive people: www.poz.com/.
- *Positively Aware.* A magazine for HIV-positive people, that includes updates on drug development and scientific developments : www.tpan.com/.
- *Project Inform.* An organization that provides updated information about HIV treatment. www.projinf.org/.

Glossary

A

Abscesses: Collections of pus (infectious organisms and white blood cells) in the skin ("boil") or other parts of the body.

Acquired immunodeficiency syndrome: See "AIDS."

Acute retroviral syndrome (ARS): A collection of symptoms, such as fever, rash, and swollen lymph nodes, which most people experience during primary infection, shortly after they're infected.

Acyclovir (*Zovirax*): A drug used to treat herpes simplex and varicella zoster virus.

ADAP: See "AIDS Drug Assistance Program."

Adherence: The term used to refer to a patient's behavior with respect to following treatment recommendations, including taking medications, keeping medical appointments, etc.

Adrenal gland: A gland in the abdomen that produces cortisol, a steroid hormone that is essential to many bodily functions, including the response to stress.

Adrenal insufficiency: A deficiency in the amount of cortisol produced by the adrenal gland.

Advance directives: Legal documents that allow you to make decisions about end-of-life care ahead of time. See "Living Will" and "Durable Power of Attorney for Health Care."

Advanced HIV infection: The most advanced stage of HIV infection, usually in people with CD4 counts below 50 or 100.

Aerosolized pentamidine: See "pentamidine."

AIDS: Acquired immunodeficiency syndrome, a more advanced stage of HIV infection, defined by having a CD4 count below 200 or one of a list of AIDS indicator conditions (see Table 1).

AIDS case definition: The criteria used by the Centers for Disease Control (CDC) to classify someone as having AIDS (see "AIDS").

AIDS-defining condition: See "AIDS-indicator condition."

AIDS Drug Assistance Program (ADAP): A federally funded program that provides antiretroviral medications and other HIV-related medications to those who have no other way to pay for them. The programs are administered by the states, and coverage varies from state to state.

AIDS-indicator condition (or AIDS-defining condition): One of a list of conditions, including opportunistic infections and malignancies, that is used by the CDC to determine who has AIDS (see Table 1).

AIDS-related complex (ARC): An old term, no longer in use, for the stage of HIV disease in which people have symptoms but have not yet developed AIDS. Now referred to as "symptomatic HIV infection."

AIDS service organization: An organization that provides services to people with HIV infection.

Alpha-fetoprotein (AFP): A blood test used to look for liver cancer.

Alternative medicine: The use of a non-standard medical treatment in place of standard therapy.

Amphotericin B: An intravenous drug used to treat serious fungal infections.

Anal cancer: A cancer of the anus caused by human papillomavirus (HPV).

Anal dysplasia: Abnormal cells in the anus caused by human papillomavirus (HPV). If left untreated, it can progress to anal cancer.

Anal Pap smears: A diagnostic test to screen for anal dysplasia.

Anemia: A deficiency of red blood cells, usually diagnosed by a low hemoglobin or hematocrit on a complete blood count.

Angular cheilitis: Cracking of the corners of the lips, sometimes caused by Candida.

Anoscopy: See "high resolution anoscopy."

Anti-HBs: See "HBsAb."

Antibodies: Proteins used by the immune system to fight infection. Antibodies are formed after exposure to antigens, foreign substances such as viruses or bacteria.

Antidepressant: Drugs used to treat depression.

Antigens: Proteins from organisms, such as bacteria or viruses, that stimulate an immune response.

Antiretroviral therapy (ART): Drug therapy that stops HIV from replicating and improves the function of the immune system.

Anti-CMV IgG: A blood test used to look for infection with CMV.

Anti-*Toxoplasma* IgG antibody test: A blood test used to look for exposure to the *Toxoplasma* parasite.

Aphthous ulcers: Painful ulcers in the mouth (**aphthous stomatitis**) or esophagus (**aphthous esophagitis**) that can occur in people with HIV. The cause is unknown.

ARC: See "AIDS-related complex."

ART: See "antiretroviral therapy."

Aseptic meningitis: Meningitis that is not caused by a bacterium that can be grown in culture. Can be caused by viruses (including HIV during acute retroviral syndrome) or drugs.

Aspergillus: A fungus that causes aspergillosis, a potentially serious infection involving the lungs that can occur in people with very advanced HIV disease.

Asymptomatic HIV infection: An early stage of HIV infection in which infected people have a positive test but no symptoms.

Atovaquone (*Mepron*): A drug used to treat or prevent PCP.

Attachment: The first stage of entry, in which the virus binds to the CD4 receptor. Attachment inhibitors would block this step, though none are currently approved.

Avascular necrosis: Painful joint damage caused by osteonecrosis, usually affecting the hips but sometimes the shoulders.

Azithromycin: An antibiotic that can be used to treat or prevent MAC as well as some bacterial lung infections.

B

Bacillary angiomatosis: A skin bacterial disease caused by Bartonella, which causes raised purple lesions on the skin sometimes confused with Kaposi's sarcoma.

Bacterial vaginosis: A bacterial infection of the vagina that causes vaginal discharge.

Bactrim: See "trimethoprim-sulfamethoxazole."

Bartonella: The bacterium that cause peliosis hepatis and bacillary angiomatosis.

Bell's palsy: A paralysis of one side of the face that can be caused by a variety of infections, including acute HIV infection.

Benzodiazepine: A class of drugs used to treat anxiety and insomnia. Diazepam (*Valium*) is the best known example. The drugs can be habit-forming and can interact with some antiretroviral drugs.

Bilirubin: A pigment produced in the liver. When bilirubin levels get too high, the skin and eyes can turn yellow ("jaundice" or "icterus"). Elevated bilirubin can be caused by hepatitis or by two antiretroviral drugs: indinavir (*Crixivan*) or atazanavir (*Reyataz*).

Biopsy: A procedure in which a piece of tissue is removed, either with a needle through the skin, through a scope placed in the lungs or gastrointestinal tract, or by a surgical procedure. The specimen is then examined under the microscope and/or submitted for culture to make a diagnosis.

Blip: A single detectable viral load with undetectable viral loads before and after.

Boosted protease inhibitors: These combine a protease inhibitor (PI) with a low dose of ritonavir (*Norvir*), another PI that is used only to increase drug levels and prolong the half-life of other PIs.

Bronchitis: An infection of the bronchi (airways), usually caused by a viral infection often after a common cold.

Bronchoscopy: A diagnostic procedure in which a flexible tube is inserted into the lungs through the mouth (under sedation) so that samples or biopsies can be taken.

Bronchospasm: The tendency of the bronchi (airways in the lung) to constrict (narrow), causing shortness of breath or cough. This can be chronic (in patients with asthma, for example) or temporary, following an upper respiratory infection.

Burkitt's lymphoma: A type of lymphoma that is seen more frequently in people with HIV infection but is less common than non-Hodgkin's lymphoma (NHL).

C

Candida: A fungus (yeast) that can cause thrush, esophagitis, and vaginitis in people with HIV infection.

Candidiasis: An infection caused by *Candida*.

Case manager: A person who helps coordinate your medical care, provides referrals for needed services, and determines whether you qualify for any assistance or entitlement programs. A case manager is often, but not always, a social worker.

CBC: See "complete blood count."

CCR5: See "coreceptor."

CCR5 antagonists: A drug that blocks CCR5.

CD4 cell: See "CD4 lymphocyte."

CD4 cell count: See "CD4 count."

CD4 count (or CD4 cell count): A lab test that measures the number of CD4 cells in the blood (expressed as number of cells per cubic millimeter). The CD4 count is the most important measure of immunosuppression and is the most important indicator of the need for treatment.

CD4 lymphocyte (or CD4 cell, or T-helper cell): A type of lymphocyte (a type of white blood cell) that can be infected by HIV. CD4 cells fight certain infections and cancers. The number of CD4 cells (CD4 count) declines with untreated HIV infection, which leads to immunosuppression.

CD4 percent: The percentage of lymphocytes that are CD4 cells. The CD4 percent is provided whenever a CD4 count is ordered and provides additional information about the state of the immune system.

CD4 receptor: A protein on the surface of the CD4 cell that the virus attaches to before entering the cell.

CD8 cells (or CD8 lymphocytes, or T-suppressor cells): Another type of lymphocyte affected by HIV infection. Measuring CD8 cells is not necessary as the CD8 count is not used to make treatment decisions.

CD8 lymphocytes: See "CD8 cells."

CDC: See "Centers for Disease Control and Prevention."

Cellular immune system: The part of the immune system most directly affected by HIV infection. It controls a variety of bacterial, viral, fungal, and parasitic infections.

Centers for Disease Control and Prevention (CDC): A branch of the federal government, within the Department of Health and Human Services (DHHS) that is charged with tracking, preventing, and controlling health problems in the United States, including infectious diseases such as HIV.

Cervical cancer: A cancer of the cervix (the mouth of the uterus) caused by human papillomavirus (HPV).

Cervical dysplasia: Abnormal cells of the cervix, the mouth of the uterus, caused by human papillomavirus (HPV). If left untreated, it can progress to cervical cancer.

Chemokines: See "coreceptors."

Chickenpox: See "varicella."

Chlamydia: A sexually transmitted infection caused by *Chlamydia trachomatis*.

Cholesterol: A substance found in body tissues and the blood. Cholesterol is ingested (in meat or animal products) and also manufactured by the body. Cholesterol levels are measured by blood tests.

Cirrhosis: A form of permanent liver damage caused by alcoholism or chronic hepatitis.

Clarithromycin: An antibiotic that can be used to treat or prevent MAC as well as some bacterial lung infections.

Clinical trial: A study in which a treatment for a medical condition is tested in human volunteers to determine the safety and/or effectiveness of the treatment. In the case of HIV, this could include the study of investigational or approved drugs. In a **randomized** trial, two or more treatments are compared, and the treatment is selected by random chance. In a **double-blind** trial, neither the subject nor the investigator knows which treatment the subject is receiving. In a **placebo-controlled trial**, a drug is compared against an inactive substance that is identical in appearance. In a **multicenter trial**, the same trial is conducted simultaneously at multiple centers, sometimes in multiple countries. **Phase I trials** evaluate safety and drug levels and help to determine a dose range in a small number of volunteers who may be HIV-positive or negative. **Phase II trials** are conducted in a larger number of subjects, looking at both safety and effectiveness, often of several doses of the medication. **Phase III trials** are large studies conducted at multiple sites that are designed to find out whether the treatment is effective and to collect more safety information. **Phase IV trials** occur after a treatment is already approved to find out more about its effectiveness, safety, and the best way to use it.

Clotrimazole troches: Antifungal lozenges used to treat thrush.

CMV: See "cytomegalovirus."

Coccidioidomycosis ("cocci"): A disease caused by *Coccidioides immitis*, a fungus found mostly in the deserts and valleys of the southwestern United States and northern Mexico. It can cause lung disease, meningitis, and infection of other organs.

Cocktail: A common term for an antiretroviral regimen (combination of antiretroviral drugs).

Coformulation: Two or more drugs combined into a single tablet or capsule.

Coinfection: The combination of two infections, such as HIV plus either hepatitis B virus or hepatitis C virus.

Colitis: Infection or inflammation of the colon (large intestine).

Colonization: The presence in the body of micro-organisms (viruses, bacteria, etc.) that are not causing symptoms or disease.

Colonoscopy: A medical procedure in which a flexible scope is inserted into the rectum and colon through the anus, while the patient is sedated, in order to look for abnormalities and take biopsies.

Colposcopy: A procedure used to more closely examine the cervix for dysplasia due to human papillomavirus (HPV) infection in women who have had abnormal Pap smears.

Combination therapy: The use of more than one antiretroviral drug to suppress HIV infection. All HAART is combination therapy, but not all combination therapy is HAART.

Complete blood count (CBC): A standard blood test that measures the red and white blood cell counts, hematocrit, hemoglobin, and platelet count.

Complementary and alternative medicine (CAM): Medical products or treatments that are not standard of care (see "alternative medicine" and "complementary medicine").

Complementary medicine: The use of a non-standard medical treatment in addition to standard therapy.

Compliance: See "adherence."

Comprehensive chemistry panel: A standard blood test that measures kidney function, looks for evidence of liver disease, assesses nutritional status, and looks for electrolyte (sodium, potassium) abnormalities.

Coreceptors (or chemokines): Proteins on the surface of the CD4 cell and other cells that the virus binds to after attaching to the CD4 receptor but before entering the cell. There are two coreceptors: CCR5 and CXCR4.

Cortisol: The steroid hormone produced by the adrenal gland essential to many bodily functions, including the response to stress.

Cotrimoxazole: See "trimethoprim-sulfamethoxazole."

CPR: Cardiopulmonary resuscitation. Procedures used to try to revive someone whose heart has stopped and/or has stopped breathing.

Cross-resistance: Resistance to one drug that results in resistance to other drugs, usually in the same class.

Cryptococcal antigen: A lab test performed on either blood or spinal fluid used to diagnose cryptococcal meningitis.

Cryptococcal meningitis: Meningitis (infection of the spinal fluid and spinal cord lining) caused by *Cryptococcus*.

Cryptococcus: A fungus or yeast that is a common cause of meningitis in people with HIV infection.

Cryptosporidiosis: Diarrhea caused by *Cryptosporidium*, a parasite that can be found in contaminated water or transmitted from person to person.

Cushing's syndrome: Excessive cortisol levels either because of overproduction by the adrenal glands or use of steroid medications.

CXCR4: See "coreceptors."

Cytomegalovirus (CMV): A virus that can infect the eyes, the gastrointestinal tract, the liver, and the nervous system in people with advanced HIV. The most common cause of retinitis (infection of the back of the eye).

D

Dapsone: A drug used to treat or prevent PCP and to prevent toxoplasmosis.

Daraprim: See "pyrimethamine."

Detectable: A word used to describe a viral load that is high enough to be measured by a viral load test. A detectable viral load is one that is above 50 to 400, depending on which test is being used.

Detoxification: The removal of toxic substances from the body. An important function of the liver and kidneys.

Diabetes: A disorder resulting in elevated amounts of glucose (sugar) in the blood and urine.

Directly observed therapy (DOT): A program in which treatment is given to a patient directly by a healthcare professional, at home or in a clinic, in order to ensure that it's taken. Most common with treatment for tuberculosis but sometimes used for HIV therapy.

DNA: Deoxyribonucleic acid, the genetic material of humans and most other life forms. There is no DNA in the HIV virus, but its RNA can be turned into DNA by reverse transcriptase.

Drug classes: Categories or groups of HIV drugs that are determined by the way the drugs work and the stage of the viral life cycle that they targets.

Drug holiday: The term for an interruption in therapy when the decision has been made by the patient.

dT: See "tetanus toxoid."

Durable Power of Attorney for Health Care: A legal document that allows you to authorize someone else to make medical decisions on your behalf if you loose the ability to make decisions for yourself.

Dysphagia: Difficulty swallowing.

Glossary

Dysplasia: Abnormal development or growth of tissues, organs, or cells.

E

EBV: See Epstein-Barr virus."

EIA: See "enzyme-linked immunoassay."

ELIA: See "enzyme-linked immunoassay."

Elite controllers: HIV-infected people whose viral loads are undetectable without treatment.

Encephalitis: An infection of the brain.

Endoscopy: A medical procedure in which a flexible tube is inserted into the esophagus and stomach through the mouth, while the patient is sedated, in order to take samples or biopsies or to treat a variety of conditions.

Enzyme-linked immunoassay (EIA or ELISA): The initial antibody test used to diagnose HIV infection. Positive tests must be confirmed, usually with a Western blot assay.

Enteritis: Infection or inflammation of the small intestines.

Entry: The process by which HIV enters human cells.

Entry inhibitors: Drugs that block entry.

Envelope: The outer surface of the HIV virus.

Enzymes: Proteins that carry out a biological function. Examples of enzymes carried by HIV include reverse transcriptase, integrase, and protease. Each plays a role in allowing the virus to reproduce, and each is a target for antiretroviral therapy.

Epidemic: The appearance of new cases of disease (especially an infectious disease) in a human population at a higher rate than would be expected.

Epstein-Barr virus (EBV): A herpesvirus that causes infectious mononucleosis ("mono"), oral hairy leukoplakia, and some lymphomas.

Erythematous candidiasis: An infection of the mouth caused by *Candida* in which the roof of the mouth (palate) becomes red and sometimes painful.

Esophagitis: Infection or inflammation of the esophagus.

Esophagus: The tube that connects the mouth and throat to the stomach.

F

Failure: Loss of activity of ART. Includes virologic failure (detectable viral load on therapy), immunologic failure (falling CD4 count on therapy), and clinical failure (worsening symptoms on therapy).

Famciclovir (*Famvir*): A drug used to treat herpes simplex and varicella zoster virus.

Family Medical Leave Act (FMLA): A federal law that allows people to take time off work without fear of termination or loss of benefits to deal with their own serious or chronic medical problems or those of their family members. People who need this protection must file paper-work with their employers in advance.

Fat accumulation(or lipohyper trophy): A component of the "lipodystrophy syndrome" in which fat accumulates in abnormal parts of the body, such as inside the abdomen, around the neck, in the breasts, or on the upper back at the base of the neck ("buffalo hump").

"Flu:" See "influenza."

Fluconazole (*Diflucan*): A drug used to treat fungal infections.

Flucytosine (5FC, *Ancobon*): A drug used to treat fungal infections, usually in combination with amphotericin.

FMLA: See "Family Medical Leave Act."

Folinic acid: See "leucovorin."

Folliculitis: Infection of the hair follicles and skin around them.

Fusion: The final stage of viral entry in which the envelope of the virus fuses (merges) with the membrane of the cell, allowing entry of the virus into the cells. A fusion inhibitor blocks this process.

G

Gastrointestinal: Relating to the GI tract: esophagus, stomach, small intestines, colon, and rectum.

Gastritis: Infection or inflammation of the stomach.

Genotypes: In HIV, a type of resistance test that looks for specific resistance mutations known to cause resistance to antiretroviral drugs. (See also "HCV genotype.")

Gonorrhea: A sexually transmitted infection caused by the bacterium *Neisseria gonorrheae.*

gp120: The part of the envelope (outer surface) of HIV that binds to receptors on the surface of the CD4 cell, allowing entry into the cell.

Guillain-Barré syndrome: Progressive muscle paralysis starting in the legs and moving upward, sometimes seen during acute retroviral syndrome.

H

HAART: See "highly active antiretroviral therapy."

Half-life: The amount of time it takes for the blood levels of a drug to decline by 50% after the last dose. Drugs with longer half-lives remain in the blood longer and can be taken less often.

HAV antibody: A blood test for hepatitis A. The IgM antibody tests for acute hepatitis A. The total or IgG antibody tests for prior infection or vaccination.

HBsAb (or anti-HBs): A blood test for hepatitis B. A positive result means you're immune to the hepatitis B virus either because of prior infection or vaccination.

HBsAg: A blood test for hepatitis B. A positive result means there is active hepatitis, but it doesn't distinguish between acute and chronic hepatitis.

HBV DNA: The "viral load" for hepatitis B, used to make the diagnosis in some people with negative HBV antibodies and to monitor response to hepatitis B therapy.

HCV RNA: The "viral load" for hepatitis C, used to confirm the diagnosis in people with a positive HCV antibody, to make the diagnosis in some people with a negative antibody, and to monitor response to hepatitis C therapy.

Hematocrit: A measure of the amount of red blood cells in the blood. (See "complete blood count" and "anemia.")

Hemoglobin: The oxygen-carrying component of red blood cells. Also used as a measure of the amount of red blood cells in the blood. (See "complete blood count" and "anemia.")

Hepatic steatosis ("fatty liver"): A build-up of fat in the liver that can be caused by a variety of medical conditions. When caused by antiretroviral agents it is often accompanied by lactic acidosis.

Hepatitis: Inflammation or infection of the liver.

Hepatitis A: A viral infection of the liver caused by hepatitis A virus (HAV). It is spread by ingestion of feces or of food or water contaminated by feces. Unlike hepatitis B and C, hepatitis A never causes chronic infection.

Hepatitis B: A viral infection of the liver caused by hepatitis B virus (HBV). Like HIV, it is spread sexually, through exposure to infected blood or at childbirth. A proportion of people with HBV infection can develop chronic hepatitis and liver disease.

Hepatitis C: A viral infection of the liver caused by **hepatitis C virus (HCV)**. It is spread primarily through exposure to blood (injection drug use or occupational exposures), but can also be transmitted sexually. Hepatitis C commonly causes chronic infection.

Hepatocellular carcinoma (or hepatoma, or liver cancer): A cancer of the liver that can be caused by alcoholism or chronic hepatitis.

Hepatoma: See "hepatocellular carcinoma."

Hepatotoxicity: See "liver toxicity."

Herpes simplex virus (HSV): A virus that causes painful blisters and ulcers on the lips, genitals, near the anus, or other parts of the skin. **HSV-1** is a common cause of **herpes labialis** ("cold sores") on the lips. **HSV-2** is more likely to affect the genitals or anus.

Herpesvirus: A family of viruses that can cause acute infection but that also remain latent in the body and recur. Examples of herpesviruses include herpes simplex virus (HSV), varicella zoster virus (VZV), cytomegalovirus (CMV), Epstein-Barr virus (EBV), and human herpesvirus-8 (HHV-8).

Herpes zoster: See "shingles."

HHV-8: The virus that causes Kaposi's sarcoma, Castleman's syndrome, and some rare lymphomas. Also called Kaposi's sarcoma-associated herpesvirus (KSHV).

Highly active antiretroviral therapy (HAART): Antiretroviral therapy meant to suppress the viral load to undetectable levels, using a combination of several agents to prevent resistance.

High resolution anoscopy (HRA): A procedure used to more closely examine the lining of the anus for dysplasia due to human papillomavirus (HPV) infection in people who have had abnormal anal Pap smears.

Histoplasmosis: A disease caused by *Histoplasma capsulatum*, a fungus found mostly in the Ohio and Mississippi River valleys, which causes lung infection in people with normal immune systems, and infection of the lungs and other organs in people with low CD4 counts.

HIV: Human immunodeficiency virus, the virus that causes HIV infection and AIDS.

HIVAN: See "nephropathy, HIV-associated."

HIV-1: The most common form of HIV worldwide.

HIV infection (or HIV disease): The name for the disease caused by HIV infection. "AIDS" is a late stage of HIV infection.

HLA B*5701: A blood test used to predict the likelihood of the abacavir hypersensitivity reaction (HSR). If the test is positive, you shouldn't take abacavir. If it's negative, you're unlikely to develop HSR.

Hodgkin's disease: A type of lymphoma that is more common in people with HIV but is less common than non-Hodgkin's lymphoma (NHL).

Home tests: An HIV blood test that can be used at home. Blood is put on a piece of filter paper and returned by mail. The results are then provided over the phone. The only approved home test is currently the *Home Access* test.

HPV: See "human papillomavirus."

HRA: See "high resolution anoscopy."

HSRs: See "hypersensitivity reactions."

Human herpesvirus-8: See "HHV-8."

Human immunodeficiency virus: See "HIV."

Human papillomavirus (HPV): A sexually transmitted virus that causes abnormal cells (dysplasia) in the cervix, anus, and mouth, which can lead to cancer if not treated.

Humoral immune system: The part of the immune system that uses antibodies to fight infection. It is less affected by HIV infection than the cellular immune system.

Hypersensitivity reactions (HSRs): Reactions, often allergic, to a medication or other substance.

Hypogonadism: A deficiency of testosterone, the male sex hormone.

Hypothyroidism: A deficiency in thyroid hormone.

I

Immune activation: A general stimulation of the immune system that can be caused by a variety of infections, in-

Glossary

cluding HIV infection. In the case of HIV, it is thought to cause the decline in CD4 count that occurs with time.

Immune-based therapy: Treatment for HIV infection designed to affect the immune system and its response to the virus, as opposed to standard antiretroviral therapy, which suppresses the virus itself.

Immune system: The system in the body that fights infection.

Immunodeficiency (or immunosuppression): A state in which the immune system is damaged or impaired, either from birth (congenital immunodeficiency) or acquired, as in HIV infection.

Immune reconstitution inflammatory syndrome (IRIS): A condition that sometimes occurs in people with low CD4 counts who start ART in which the improved immune system reacts to organisms (such as MAC, the TB bacterium, or fungi), causing illness, including fevers, weight loss, swollen lymph nodes, or abscesses.

Indeterminate HIV serology: This occurs when the EIA is positive but the Western blot contains some bands that are seen with HIV infection, though not enough to make a diagnosis. This can occur during the process of seroconversion or it can be found in uninfected people, usually for unclear reasons.

Induced sputum: A test used to diagnose PCP or tuberculosis in which patients inhale a saline mist that makes them cough deeply. The sputum speci-

men is then sent to the lab for analysis. Also called "sputum induction."

Influenza ("flu"): A viral infection caused by influenza virus that causes fever, muscle aches, respiratory symptoms, and gastrointestinal symptoms during winter months and should be prevented by vaccination in the fall. A bad cold is not the flu.

INH: See "isoniazid."

Insulin resistance: A condition in which the body cannot respond to insulin as well as it should. This applies both to insulin naturally produced by the pancreas and insulin injected as medication. Can lead to high blood sugar or diabetes.

Integrase: A viral enzyme that allows integration (insertion) of viral DNA into human DNA. An integrase inhibitor is an antiretroviral drug that blocks this process.

Integration: The insertion of viral DNA into human DNA in the nucleus of the cell.

Interferon: An injectable medication used to treat hepatitis C and sometimes hepatitis B.

Interferon-gamma releasing assay (IGRA): A blood test used to detect latent infection with the TB bacterium as an alternative to a tuberculin skin test.

IRIS: See "immune reconstitution inflammatory syndrome."

Isosporiasis: A disease caused by the parasite *Isospora belli*, which causes chronic diarrhea in people with low

CD4 counts. Uncommon in the United States and other developed countries.

Isoniazid (INH): A drug used to treat or prevent tuberculosis.

J

JC virus: The cause of progressive multifocal leukoencephalopathy (PML).

K

Kaposi's sarcoma (KS): A tumor caused by a virus that is more common in people with HIV infection, especially gay men. Although it usually affects the skin, KS can also affect other parts of the body, including the gastrointestinal tract and lungs.

Kaposi's sarcoma-associated herpesvirus (KSHV): See "HHV-8."

Kidney biopsy: A procedure in which a piece of a kidney is removed using a needle inserted through the skin in order to find out the cause of kidney disorders.

Koch's postulates: The four criteria needed to prove that a microbe or organism is the cause of a disease. The postulates are: 1. The organism must be found in all animals suffering from the disease but should not be found in healthy animals; 2. The organism must be isolated from a diseased animal and grown in pure culture; 3. The cultured organism should cause disease when introduced into a healthy animal; and 4. The organism must be reisolated from the experimentally infected animal.

KS: See "Kaposi's sarcoma."

KSHV: See "Kaposi's sarcoma-associated herpesvirus."

L

Lactic acidosis: A dangerous build-up of lactic acid (lactate) in the blood, which can be caused by some antiretroviral drugs and also by other medical conditions.

Latency: The ability of HIV to persist in human cells for the lifetime of an infected individual by inserting its DNA into long-lived reservoir cells.

Leukopenia: A decrease in the number of white blood cells found in blood.

Leucovorin (folinic acid): A drug used to prevent bone marrow toxicity due to pyrimethamine.

LGV: See "lymphogranuloma venereum."

Life cycle: In HIV infection, the stages that the virus goes through, starting with its entry into human cells and ending with its replication and the release of new virus particles into the blood.

Lipoatrophy: Loss of subcutaneous fat (fat under the skin) in the legs, arms, buttocks, and face, caused by some nucleoside analog reverse transcriptase inhibitors (NRTIs).

Lipodystrophy: A general term for changes in body shape and fat distribution caused by some antiretroviral agents. Can include lipoatrophy, fat accumulation, or both.

Lipohypertrophy: See "fat accumulation."

Listeria: A foodborne bacterium that can cause meningitis and other infections. Although not common, the risk for acquiring *Listeria* is higher in people with HIV.

Liver biopsy: The removal of a piece of the liver for diagnostic purposes, either with a needle inserted through the skin, or by a catheter inserted into a vein.

Liver cancer: See "hepatocellular carcinoma."

Liver enzymes: See "transaminases."

Liver toxicity (or hepatotoxicity): Damage to the liver caused by medications.

Living Will: A legal document that allows you to state which medical procedures and life-sustaining measures you would want if you were no longer able to make decisions for yourself.

Log (logarithm): Another way of expressing viral load results. A viral load of 100,000 is a viral load of five logs; 10,000 is four logs; 1,000 is three logs. A tenfold change in viral load is a one-log change. For example, a drop in viral load from 100,000 to 1,000 is a "two-log drop."

Lumbar puncture: See "spinal tap."

Lymphadenopathy: Swollen or enlarged lymph nodes ("glands"). (See also "persistent generalized lymphadenopathy.")

Lymph nodes: Structures of the human body that are part of the immune system, acting as filters that collect and destroy bacteria and viruses.

Lymphocytes: A type of infection-fighting white blood cell. CD4 cells are a type of lymphocyte.

Lymphogranuloma venereum (LGV): A sexually transmitted infection caused by *Chlamydia*.

Lymphoma: A cancer of the lymphatic tissue that is more common in people with HIV infection. Can occur in virtually any part of the body.

M

MAC: See "*Mycobacterium avium* complex."

MAI: See "*Mycobacterium avium* complex."

Medicaid: An insurance program funded by the federal and state governments that provides coverage for medical care to low-income, uninsured people.

Medicare: A federally funded program to provide medical insurance primarily to the elderly and disabled.

Meningitis: An infection or inflammation of the spinal fluid and the lining of the spinal cord.

Methicillin-resistant *Staphylococcus aureus* (MRSA): A drug-resistant bacterium that traditionally caused serious illness in seriously ill hospitalized patients but that has recently become a common cause of skin disease, including abscesses (community-acquired MRSA).

Microsporidia: A variety of opportunistic parasites with hard-to-pronounce names that change frequently. They can cause chronic diarrhea in people with low CD4 counts.

Migraine headache: A severe headache, often on one side of the head, sometimes accompanied by visual changes or nausea.

Molluscum contagiosum: Flesh-colored bumps or protuberances on the skin that are caused by a poxvirus and can be sexually transmitted.

MRSA: See "methicillin-resistant *Staphylococcus aureus.*"

Mucosal c ells: Cells that line the internal organs and body orifices, such as the mouth, nostrils, anus, and genital area.

Mutation: Changes in the normal genetic make-up of an organism due to a mistake that occurs during reproduction. In the case of HIV, some mutations can cause resistance, allowing the virus to replicate in the presence of antiretroviral drugs.

***Mycobacterium avium* complex (MAC):** A bacterium related to tuberculosis that causes disease in people with advanced HIV disease, including fever, night sweats, weight loss, diarrhea, liver disease, abdominal pain, and anemia. Also known as *Mycobacterium avium intracellulare* (MAI).

Myelitis: Infection or inflammation of the spinal cord.

Myopathy: An inflammation of muscles causing muscle pain and weakness, sometimes seen with acute retroviral syndrome, high-dose zidovudine, or "statins" used to lower cholesterol.

N

National Institutes of Health (NIH): An agency of the federal government (under the Department of Health and Human Services) responsible for conducting and funding medical research.

Nephropathy, HIV-associated (HIVAN): A disease of the kidneys caused by HIV infection. It is seen almost only in black patients.

Neuropathy (or peripheral neuropathy): Damage to the nerves resulting in numbness or burning pain, usually in the feet or legs. Can be caused by HIV, some antiretroviral drugs, or other conditions.

Neuropsychological testing: A series of tests, usually performed by a psychologist or neurologist, to assess memory and thinking skills. Can be used to diagnose dementia, or to determine whether someone has depression or dementia.

NHL: See "non-Hodgkin's lymphoma."

NIH: See "National Institutes of Health."

NNRTIs: See "non-nucleoside reverse transcriptase inhibitors."

Non-Hodgkin's lymphoma (NHL): The most common type of lymphoma in people with HIV infection.

Non-nucleoside reverse transcriptase inhibitors (NNRTIs): A class of antiretroviral drugs that blocks reverse transcription of viral RNA into DNA by interfering with the activity of reverse transcriptase.

Non-steroidal anti-inflammatory drugs (NSAIDs): Drugs that are commonly used to suppress inflammation and treat pain. Some are available without a prescription.

NRTIs: See "nucleoside analog reverse transcriptase inhibitors."

NSAIDs: See "non-steroidal anti-inflammatory drugs."

Nucleoside analog reverse transcriptase inhibitors (NRTIs or "nukes"): A class of antiretroviral drugs that blocks reverse transcription of viral RNA into DNA by mimicking nucleosides, the normal building blocks of DNA.

"Nukes:" See "nucleoside analog reverse transcriptase inhibitors."

Nystatin: An antifungal mouth rinse used to treat thrush.

O

Odynophagia: Painful swallowing.

OI: See "opportunistic infections."

Opportunistic infections (OIs): Infections that takes advantage of immunodeficiency. Some opportunistic infections occur *only* in people who are immunosuppressed; others can occur in anyone but are more severe or progressive with immunosuppression.

Oral hairy leukoplakia (OHL): Painless white plaques, or "stripes," on the sides of the tongue caused by Epstein-Barr virus.

Oropharyngeal candidiasis: *Candida* (yeast) infection involving the mouth and throat, including thrush, angular cheilitis, and erythematous candidiasis.

Osteonecrosis: Damage to bones at the large joints. See "avascular necrosis."

Osteopenia: A loss of bone density ("thinning of the bones").

Osteoporosis: Severe osteopenia, which can lead to bone fractures.

P

Pancreas: An organ in the abdomen that makes insulin and enzymes that help digest food.

Pancreatitis: Inflammation of the pancreas, resulting in abdominal pain, loss of appetite, nausea, and vomiting. Can be fatal.

Pandemic: A global epidemic.

Pap smear: A diagnostic test used to look for cervical dysplasia and cervical cancer. Now also being used to diagnose anal dysplasia (See "anal Pap smear").

Pathogen: An infectious organism (bacterium, virus, fungus, or parasite) that causes disease.

PCNSL: See "primary central nervous system lymphoma."

PCP: : Used to stand for *Pneumocystis carinii* pneumonia, one of the most common OIs in an HIV-positive patient. See "*Pneumocystis*."

PCR: See "polymerase chain reaction."

Pegylated interferon: The preferred form of interferon, as it can be injected less frequently and has fewer side effects.

Peliosis hepatis: An uncommon bacterial liver infection caused by *Bartonella*.

Pelvic inflammatory disease (PID): A serious infection of the uterus and fallopian tubes usually caused by sexually transmitted infections, especially gonorrhea and chlamydia.

Pentamidine: A drug used to treat PCP. Aerosolized pentamidine is used as an inhaled mist to prevent PCP.

Perinatal transmission: Transmission of HIV from mother to infant during late pregnancy, labor, or breastfeeding.

Peripheral neuropathy: See "neuropathy."

Pharynx: Throat.

Phenotypes: A type of resistance test that measures the ability of the virus to replicate in varying concentrations of antiretroviral drugs.

PID: See "pelvic inflammatory disease."

Plasma HIV RNA: See "viral load."

Platelets: Blood cells that helps blood clot. A low platelet count, which can sometimes occur due to HIV infection, can result in easy bleeding or bruising.

PML: See "progressive multifocal leukoencephalopathy."

Pneumococcal polysaccharide vaccine (*Pneumovax*): A vaccine recommended for HIV-positive adults to prevent pneumonia caused by the pneumococcus.

Pneumococcus: The common name for *Streptococcus pneumoniae*, a frequent cause of bacterial pneumonia.

Pneumocystis: A fungus (*Pneumocystis jiroveci*) that is a common cause of pneumonia (PCP) in people with HIV infection.

Pneumonia: An infection of the air spaces of the lungs, which can be caused by a variety of infectious organisms.

Pneumovax: See "pneumococcal polysaccharide vaccine."

Polymerase chain reaction (PCR): A laboratory technique used to detect or quantify the DNA or RNA of an infectious organism for diagnostic purposes.

PPD: See "tuberculin skin test."

Pre-exposure prophylaxis (PrEP): The use of antiretroviral drugs by HIV-negative people to prevent infection.

PrEP: See "pre-exposure prophylaxis."

Primary central nervous system lymphoma (PCNSL): A lymphoma involving the brain, seen only in people with advanced HIV disease.

Primary HIV infection: The stage of HIV infection that occurs shortly after infection. At this stage, the viral load is very high but antibody tests may be negative or indeterminate. People often have symptoms during this stage (See "acute retroviral syndrome").

Proctitis: Infection or inflammation of the anus and rectum.

Progressive multifocal leukoencephalopathy (PML): An infection of the brain caused by JC virus, which results in progressive neurologic deterioration.

Prophylaxis: Prevention, usually applied to the use of medications taken to prevent opportunistic infections or to keep them from coming back after they've been treated.

Protease: A viral enzyme that cuts large viral proteins into smaller proteins, which are then used to create new virus particles. A protease inhibitor (PI) is an antiretroviral drug that blocks this process.

Prurigo nodularis: A condition characterized by itchy bumps on the skin, seen more commonly in people with HIV.

Psoriasis: A skin condition that results in dry, scaly, itchy plaques on the skin that can get worse with immunosuppression due to HIV infection.

Purified protein derivative (PPD): See "tuberculin skin test."

Pyrimethamine (*Daraprim*): A drug used to treat or prevent PCP or toxoplasmosis.

R

R5 virus: HIV that enters the CD4 cell using the CCR5 coreceptor. This type of virus can be treated with CCR5 inhibitors. (See also "coreceptor.")

Radiculitis (radiculopathy): Infection or inflammation of the nerves that emerge from the spinal cord.

Rapid tests: HIV tests that provide an answer within a few minutes, using either blood or saliva. Positive tests must be confirmed with standard serologies.

Reactive airways: See "bronchospasm."

Recombinant strains: Strains of HIV that are combinations of two or more other strains.

Red blood cell (RBC): Blood cells that carry oxygen to the organs of the body. If you don't have enough of them, you're anemic.

Regimen: A combination of antiretroviral drugs.

Relapse: The return of an illness or disease, usually in someone with a chronic condition.

Replication: The reproduction or multiplication of an organism, including HIV. The replication of HIV is a complex, multi-step process involving infection of a human cell and use of both viral enzymes and human cellular machinery to create new virus particles, which are then released and can infect new cells.

Reservoir: Long-lived human cells that can be infected by HIV, allowing it to persist (remain latent) for the lifetime of the individual. Resting CD4 cells are the best known example, but there are other reservoirs in the human body.

Resistance: The ability of the virus to replicate despite the presence of antiretroviral medications.

Resistance test: A blood test (either a genotype or phenotype) that looks for evidence in the presence of HIV that is resistant to antiretroviral medications.

Resting CD4 cells: CD4 cells that live a long time and can harbor HIV DNA, which can't be affected by antiretroviral therapy because it's not replicating. An important reservoir of latent HIV.

Retinitis: An infection of the retina (the interior surface of the back of the eye) which can lead to blindness if not treated. Most often caused by CMV.

Retrovirus: A virus that contains RNA and that can turn RNA into DNA through reverse transcription using viral enzymes. (See "reverse transcription.") HIV is a retrovirus.

Reverse transcriptase (RT): An enzyme contained within the HIV virus that can turn viral RNA into DNA so it can be inserted into the DNA of human cells. A reverse transcriptase inhibitor blocks this process.

Reverse transcription: The conversion of viral RNA into DNA by reverse transcriptase. (Normal transcription involves the conversion of DNA into RNA.)

Rifabutin: A drug used to treat or prevent MAC. It is also used as an alternative to rifampin to treat tuberculosis.

Rifampin: A drug used to treat tuberculosis and some other bacterial infections.

RNA: Ribonucleic acid, the genetic material of the HIV virus. Viral RNA gets turned into DNA by reverse transcriptase, and the viral DNA then gets inserted into the DNA of human cells. DNA is later transcribed back into RNA, which in turn gets translated into the proteins that are used to make new virus particles.

RT: See "reverse transcriptase."

Ryan White Care Act: A government-funded program that provides money on a state or local level to provide care for uninsured people with HIV infection.

S

Salmonella: A group of bacteria that can cause severe diarrhea, fever, and bloodstream infections.

Scabies: An itchy skin condition caused by a mite that burrows under the skin and can be spread to others by close contact.

Seborrheic dermatitis: A common skin condition causing flakiness on the face, especially around the eyebrows and in the folds on the cheeks.

Septra: See "trimethoprim-sulfamethoxazole."

Seroconversion: The process of developing an antibody to an infectious agent. In the case of HIV, it occurs shortly after primary infection.

Serologies: Blood tests that measures antibodies to look for evidence of a disease. The standard HIV test is a serology.

Sexually transmitted infections (STIs): Infections transmitted from person to person through sexual activity. Also "sexually transmitted diseases (STDs)."

Shingles (herpes zoster): A painful, blistering rash, usually occurring in a band on one side of the body, caused by reactivation of the chickenpox virus (varicella zoster virus, VZV).

Side effects: Undesirable effects of a medication or treatment that are noticeable to the person being treated. See also "toxicity."

Sinus headache: A headache caused by congestion of the sinuses. See also "sinusitis."

Sinusitis: An infection of the sinuses; air spaces in the head connected to the nasal passages.

Social Security Disability Insurance (SSDI): A monthly Social Security benefit for disabled people who have worked in the past and have paid a minimum amount of Social Security taxes.

Sperm washing: A technique in which sperm are separated from semen to lower the risk of HIV transmission to a woman during conception.

Spinal tap (lumbar puncture): A procedure in which a needle is inserted into the back between the vertebrae to collect a sample of cerebrospinal fluid (CSF) to diagnose meningitis. (Not as bad as it sounds.)

SSDI: See "Social Security Disability Insurance."

SSI: See "Supplemental Security Income."

Statins: The common name for HMG CoA reductase inhibitors, drugs that lower cholesterol.

STIs: See "sexually transmitted infections."

Strain: In the case of HIV, a type of virus, as in "drug-resistant strain."

Strep throat: The common term for streptococcal pharyngitis, a bacterial infection of the throat caused by group A beta-hemolytic *Streptococcus*.

Structured treatment interruption: The term for an interruption in therapy that's been approved by the provider.

Subcutaneous fat: Fat found under the skin.

Sub-types: In the case of HIV, groups of related viruses, also called "clades" or "sub-clades." Most HIV-positive people in the United States are infected with subtype B, but there are many other subtypes throughout the world.

Superinfection: Reinfection with a new strain of HIV in someone who has already been infected.

Supplemental Security Income (SSI): A federal cash assistance program designed to help the aged, blind, and disabled who have little or no income to pay for basic necessities.

Suppressor cell: See "CD8 cell."

Symptomatic HIV infection: A stage of HIV infection in which people have symptoms caused by HIV, such as weight loss, diarrhea, or thrush, but have not yet developed an AIDS indicator condition.

Syndrome: A collection of signs or symptoms that frequently occur together but that may or may not be caused by a single disease. AIDS was referred to as a syndrome before its cause, HIV infection, had been discovered.

Syphilis: A sexually transmitted infection caused by *Treponema pallidum*, a bacterium, that can cause anal, genital, or mouth lesions (primary syphilis), fever, rash, and hepatitis (secondary syphilis), or infection of the brain, spinal fluid, eyes, or ears (neurosyphilis). It can also be dormant, causing no symptoms (latent syphilis).

T

T-helper cell: See "CD4 cell."

T-suppressor cells: See "CD8 cells."

TB: See "tuberculosis."

Tdap: See "tetanus toxoid."

Tension headache: A headache caused by muscle tension.

Testosterone: The male sex hormone, which can be low in some HIV-positive men (see "hypogonadism").

Tetanus toxoid (dT or Tdap): A combination vaccine that should be received every 10 years for adults, regardless of HIV status. When you get a "tetanus shot," you either get dT (diphtheria-tetanus) or Tdap, which also includes the pertussis (whooping cough) vaccine.

Therapeutic vaccine: A vaccine given to treat an existing infection by stimulating the immune system to fight it.

Thrombocytopenia Disorder in which there is an abnormally low amount of platelets.

Thrush: Oral candidiasis, a yeast infection involving the mouth presenting with white/yellow curd-like plaques on the palate, gums, or the back of the throat.

TMP-SMX: A combination of two antibiotic drugs used to treat a wide variety of bacterial infections. See "trimethoprim-sulfamethoxazole."

Toxicity: Damage to the body caused by a drug or other substance.

Toxoplasma: A parasite (*Toxoplasma gondii*) that causes brain lesions (encephalitis) in people with HIV infection.

Toxoplasmosis: Disease caused by *Toxoplasma*.

Transaminases (liver enzymes): Blood tests used to look for damage to the liver.

Transcription: The process of turning DNA into RNA.

Treatment interruption: Stopping antiretroviral therapy. No longer in vogue.

Triglycerides: Fats that are ingested in the form of vegetable oils and animal fats.

Trimethoprim-sulfamethoxazole (TMP-SMX, co-trimoxazole, *Bactrim*, *Septra*): An antibiotic used to treat or prevent PCP and to prevent toxoplasmosis.

Tropism assay: A blood test used to find out whether your virus enters the CD4 cell using the CCR5 coreceptor (R5 virus) or the CXCR4 coreceptor (X4 virus). This test is necessary before taking a CCR5 inhibitor, which should only be used with R5 virus. The brand name of the test is *Trofile*.

Tuberculin skin test (TST): A skin test used to look for evidence of past exposure to *Mycobacterium tuberculosis*, the bacterium that causes tuberculosis. The most common form of TST is the PPD (purified protein derivative).

Tuberculosis (TB): A bacterial disease caused by *Mycobacterium tuberculosis*. TB most often causes lung disease but can affect any part of the body.

Typhoid vaccine: A vaccine to prevent typhoid fever, a bacterial infection of the blood caused by *Salmonella typhi*, sometimes acquired by travelers to developing countries.

U

Ultrasensitive viral load assay: A viral load test that measures viral load down to a lower limit of 20 to 75 copies/mL. (Standard assays measure viral load down to a lower limit of 400 copies/mL.)

Undetectable: A term used to describe a viral load that is too low to be measured by a viral load test. An undetectable viral load is below 20 to 400, depending on which test is being used.

Urinalysis: A standard lab test that looks for evidence of protein, sugar, blood, and infection in the urine.

V

Vaccine (vaccination): A substance that is given, usually by injection, but sometimes by mouth or by nasal spray, to stimulate the immune system to make antibodies against a bacterial or viral pathogen.

Vaginitis: Infection or inflammation of the vagina.

Valacyclovir (*Valtrex*): A drug used to treat herpes simplex and varicella zoster virus.

Valtrex: See "valacyclovir."

Varicella zoster virus: The virus that causes chicken pox (primary varicella) and shingles (herpes zoster).

Viral load (or plasma HIV RNA): A lab test that measures the amount of HIV RNA in the plasma (blood), expressed as "copies per milliliter." The viral load predicts the rate of progression to AIDS. It is the most important test for measuring the effectiveness of ART and also helps determine the need for treatment.

Virions: Single virus particles.

Virus: A microscopic organism composed of genetic material (DNA or RNA) inside a protein coat.

Visceral fat: Fat present inside the abdomen, around the internal organs, rather than under the skin.

W

WB: See "western blot."

WBC: See "white blood cell."

Western blot (WB): The confirmatory test used to diagnose HIV infection in people who test positive for HIV antibodies by EIA.

White blood cell (WBC): A type of blood cell that helps fight infection. CD4 cells are a type of lymphocyte, which is a type of white blood cell.

Wild-type virus: The strain of HIV that occurs "in the wild"—without the presence of antiretroviral drugs that could select for mutations. Generally a non-mutant, drug-sensitive virus.

Window period: The period between infection and formation of antibodies leading to a positive HIV test (serology). The window period usually last just a few weeks but rarely can take up to 3 to 6 months.

X

X4 virus: HIV that enters the CD4 cell using the CXCR4 coreceptor. X4 virus cannot be treated with CCR5 inhibitors. (See also "coreceptor.")

Y

Yeast: A group of micro-organisms (that can sometimes cause human infections, ranging from minor (oral thrush, vaginitis) to severe (cryptococcal meningitis). All yeasts are fungi.

Yellow fever: A serious disease caused by yellow fever virus, which is transmitted by mosquitoes and sometimes acquired by travelers to parts of Africa or Latin America.

Z

Zovirax: See "acyclovir."

Glossary

Index

Index

Rosuvastatin, 58
RPV. *See* Rilpivirine
RT. *See* Reverse transcriptase
RTV. *See* Ritonavir
Ryan White Care Act, 33
Ryan White-funded HIV specialty clinics, 29

S

Safer sexual practices, 19
Safe sex, 136, 137–138, 140
    negative partners and, 138–139
    positive partners and, 139–140
Salmonella, 17*t*, 106, 149
Saquinavir, 47*t*
Scabies, 112
Sculptra, 77
Seborrheic dermatitis, 112, 113
Secondary syphilis, rashes and, 112
Seizure medications, HIV drugs and, 58–59
Seizures, 113, 114
Self-efficacy, 54
Selzentry, 47*t*
Semen, 18, 138
Septra
    kidneys and, 81
    PCP treatment and, 91, 97
Seroconversion, 24
Serologies, 16, 17
Serostim, 78
Serum cryptococcal antigen, 113
Sexual activities, relative risk of, 137–138
Sexually transmitted diseases, 133
Sexually transmitted infections, 9, 10, 39, 139, 140–141
Sexual partners, disclosing HIV status to, 136–137
Sexual relationships, new, HIV infection and, 4
Sexual transmission, 18
    HIV-negative people and, 19–20
    HIV-positive people and, 20
    starting ART treatment and risk of, 46

Shingles (herpes zoster), 10, 17, 90*t*, 97, 100, 112
Shingles vaccine, 41
Shortness of breath, 107–108
Side effects, 63
    of efavirenz, 84–85
    living with, 55–56
    of non-nucleoside reverse transcriptase inhibitors, 74
    of nucleoside analogs, 75–76
    of protease inhibitors, 72–73
Simvastatin, 58
Sinus headaches, 113
Sinusitis, 109
Skin problems, 111–112
Smoking, osteopenia and, 82
Social Security Disability Insurance, 8
Sperm washing, 120
Spinal cord, 114
Spinal tap (lumbar puncture), 94
SQV. *See* Saquinavir
SSDI. *See* Social Security Disability Insurance
SSI. *See* Supplemental Security Income
St. John's wort, 68
Statins, HIV drugs and, 58
Stavudine, 47*t*, 53, 56
    hepatic steatosis and, 75
    lactic acidosis and, 75, 111
    lipoatrophy and, 75, 76
    metabolic toxicity and, 76
    neuropathy and, 75
    peripheral neuropathy and, 114
    toxic peripheral neuropathy and, 84
Steroids
    adrenal insufficiency and, 83
    IRIS and, 100
Steroid sprays, HIV drugs and, 58
Stigma, 3–7, 121, 136
STIs. *See* Sexually transmitted infections
Stocrin, 47*t*
Strain, 44
Strep throat, 109
Stroke, high cholesterol and, 72
Structured treatment interruptions, 63

Index